THE BANANA LADY

*And other stories of curious behaviour
and speech*

ANDREW KERTESZ

ISBN: 978-1-4251-0126-8

We at Trafford believe that it is the responsibility of us all, as both individuals and corporations, to make choices that are environmentally and socially sound. You, in turn, are supporting this responsible conduct each time you purchase a Trafford book, or make use of our publishing services. To find out how you are helping, please visit www.trafford.com/responsiblepublishing.html

Our mission is to efficiently provide the world's finest, most comprehensive book publishing service, enabling every author to experience success. To find out how to publish your book, your way, and have it available worldwide, visit us online at www.trafford.com/10510

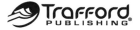

www.trafford.com

North America & international
toll-free: 1 888 232 4444 (USA & Canada)
phone: 250 383 6864 ♦ fax: 250 383 6804
email: info@trafford.com

The United Kingdom & Europe
phone: +44 (0)1865 487 395 ♦ local rate: 0845 230 9601
facsimile: +44 (0)1865 481 507 ♦ email: info.uk@trafford.com

TABLE OF CONTENTS

Foreword

These are stories about a relatively little known illness that happens to be much more common than it is generally recognized. The exact cause remains a puzzle as with many other afflictions of the nervous system, but we are beginning to understand its anatomy, genetics, and biology. It is presently classified as one of the so-called "degenerative diseases" of the brain, progressively eroding either behaviour and personality, or language and locomotion. The manifestations are often stranger than fiction, at times creating situations that strain and devastate family and social relationships.

It is commonly mistaken for Alzheimer's disease or manic-depressive illness. Many die in institutions with the wrong diagnosis and a few are diagnosed only at post-mortem. The reasons for this are many. Although it was known as a distinct clinical syndrome since Arnold Pick's description in the 19th century, its multiple clinical and pathological manifestations were and still are described as separate or rare diseases of the brain. It is a bit like the proverbial elephant. A blind sage feeling its leg may call it a tree, another feeling the body – a wall, and yet another feeling the trunk – a snake, etc. This fractionation has hampered the recognition of the illness as a relatively common entity.

This book is aimed at the lay reader interested in the brain and behaviour and the caregivers who sometimes suffer as much as the patients if not more. Technical expressions are explained when necessary. Professionals who diagnose and treat mental or neurological disease will find it useful as a case-based text. The stories are all factual, only the names of persons and places are changed. Each is chosen to represent one of the typical behaviours, but many of these are shared and recur throughout. In conjunction with each story biological, psychological and societal issues are raised, discussed, and some explanation for the behaviour is sought. Some issues are philosophical, such as what is the "self" what constitutes a personality, free will, decision making, even morality? Others are neurological, how is the brain affected and why and how the illness progresses, what forms and varieties it takes, and what is its course and inheritance? There is a concise, factual summary in lay and explained technical terms of the biology, clinical diagnosis, investigation and genetics of the disease, sufficiently informative to be useful for professionals and lay readers as well. A brief compendium of tips for caregivers is disease specific and is structured to provide a feel for the progression of problems and to provide my personal experience with coping strategies. At the end there is a glossary for the burgeoning terminology and key references to the literature.

A great deal is owed to my patients and their caregivers, who were the inspiration and source of much of the material in the book, to my administrative assistant, Bonita Stevenson, who encouraged me to write it and did the initial typing and referencing, continued by Kathy Ayers, the team of the Cognitive Neurology Unit – Wilda Davidson-Mardlin, Dr. Brian Gold, Dr. Hans Karbe, Dr. Drew Kirk, Marybelle Lozanski, Pat McCabe, Mervin Blair, Nicole Davis-Faroque, Darlyne Morlog, Koula Pantazopoulos, Dr. Cecile Marczinski, Dr Paul McMonagle and Dr. David Munoz, who worked with me and the patients while our interest and knowledge about the illness developed. I am indebted to Bonita Stevenson, Diane Wey and my wife Ann for careful editorial work, Tom Pridding for the cover art, and Connie McCann at Trafford for technical editing and design. David Munoz, a neuropathologist and neurologist, contributed substantially to our pathological conceptualizations of the disease, and co-edited the technical volume on the subject entitled, "Pick's Disease and Pick Complex" (Wiley-Liss) and the proceedings of a Frontotemporal Dementia and Pick's Disease Conference held in London, Ontario in 2002 as a supplement to the Annals of Neurology (2003).

Andrew Kertesz MD FRCP(C)
London, Ontario
June 2006

One

Introduction

IMAGINE YOURSELF IN WENCESLAS square in Prague around 1900. This should not be too difficult if you have been there recently, because this part of the city is preserved nearly as it was in its turn of the century glory. The old horse market was being replaced by one of the most elegant architectural spaces of Europe, surrounded by neorenaissance, baroque and art nouveaux apartment houses and hotels resembling palaces. The statue of the Czech King Wenceslas on horseback is to be erected in the square in front of the national museum during a time of prosperity and peace imposed by the Habsburgs. Emancipation of minorities of the empire has begun and the national capitals are undergoing rejuvenation and unprecedented growth. The square will be the scene of the "velvet" revolution 90 years later, this time against Soviet domination. Just around the corner is an elegant apartment house in Krakow st. 6, where Arnold Pick, recently appointed professor of neuropsychiatry at Charles University lives. Last time I looked it was the Bulgarian embassy and it could not be visited. Another five or so blocks south is the "new city", established by King Charles in the 14th century, where Arnold Pick taught and saw his patients in the "Katerinky", the famous Asylum of Prague on Katerinska street, now the neurological clinic. This is the backdrop to our story.

Arnold Pick described frontotemporal degeneration in a series of papers between 1892 and 1906, a new disease that was later named after him. He emphasized that progressive atrophy or shrinkage can affect the brain focally and produce the bizarre behaviour or language loss, the two distinguishing features of this condition. Until then, people had the idea of cerebral degeneration as diffuse and a consequence of aging or the "hardening of arteries" (interesting to note, the vascular causation is undergoing a major revival right now). Pick was the professor of the German department of neuropsychiatry (neurology and psychiatry separated only later, after Kraepelin and Freud). Prague was an important city of the Austro-Hungarian Empire and in earlier times in history the capital of the Holy Roman Empire, often ruled by the Habsburgs. The empire saw a reemergence of Czech nationalism in the 19th century, under the leadership of Masaryk, a contemporary of Arnold Pick at the University of Vienna. Czech deputies were given an important voice in the affairs of the country and parallel Czech departments were created at Charles University of Prague, including neuropsychiatry. Interestingly, the Czech department remained psychiatrically oriented and Pick, who was more of a neurologist, described the disease with both behavioural and language impairment. Pick had wide ranging interests in both neurology and psychiatry and he was particularly interested in the neurology of language. He wrote a book on the disturbances of grammar in association with loss of language, or aphasia. Pick's first case of the disease that later was named after him, was a man with progressive aphasia called August H. (not to be confused with Auguste D., Alzheimer's famous first patient, a woman). See the chapter "Speechless in Sarnia" for a description of primary progressive aphasia. Pick wrote: "...*The history suggests that the speech disturbance developed gradually...there was pronounced atrophy of the convolutions of the left hemisphere, particularly the left temporal lobe...*" The second publication dealt with the behavioural abnormality resembling the story of the "banana lady" and many of the others in this book. The case description is as vivid as if it had been written today: "*A 41 year old housewife changed gradually. She became careless, clumsy... did not carry out her usual work, did not take care of her children, did not change her clothes, or the bedding and stopped combing her hair. She left work unfinished and lay about idly. She did not initiate conversation, repeated questions, tended to give stereotypical answers, and often perseverated. Her only concern was her body, she complained of fleas and hunger, and was always asking for food.*"

The 19th century was a golden age of classifying diseases according to clinico-pathological observations; or in other words, to explain the symptoms observed in life, in the clinic, by looking for changes in the body postmortem. The turn of the century was especially auspicious, because of the new technology of tissue preservation with alcohol and formaldehyde and staining the brain with silver solutions to detect changes in the neurons. It was Alzheimer who described the postmortem microscopic appearance of the brain not only in the disease named after him, but also the silver staining, round, inclusions (later named Pick bodies) in cases of frontotemporal degeneration described by Pick. These "silver bullets" were declared diagnostic, but it soon became evident that only about a quarter of the patients had them at autopsy. Those who did not, were relabeled as dementia of the frontal type or frontal lobe dementia (FLD) 80 years later. The relabeling continues: recently coined terms are frontotemporal dementia (FTD), frontotemporal lobar degeneration (FTLD), primary progressive aphasia (PPA), semantic dementia (SD), or dementia lacking distinctive histology (DLDH), an awkward term that is being replaced, as most of the cases turn out to have the motor neuron disease (MND) type inclusions. This proliferation in terminology led to a confusing alphabet soup of conditions (see the glossary at the end), considered rare and unrelated. It was not until the last ten years that the relationships of these various entities are beginning to be recognized. Although the use of the term Pick's disease would be preferable to many, it is often restricted in the technical literature to the pathology with Pick bodies. This restriction resulted in the mistaken dogma that the disease is rare and in the paradox that only pathologists can diagnose it after the patient dies. One would be justified to ask: what good is it to define a disease, if you can only diagnose it in the afterlife?

David Munoz, my outstanding pathologist collaborator, and other prominent pathologists were not ready (and are still not) to give the name back to the clinicians, therefore he and I suggested the term Pick complex for the whole entity, to cut through the terminological confusion. Many use the term Frontotemporal Dementia (FTD), or Frontotemporal lobar degeneration (FTLD) for the overall condition and these terms will be used in the book interchangeably. Many dislike the term dementia, and since most of these patients only have personality change and/or language deficit initially, one could argue that they are not demented. The clinical and pathological overlap between the varieties of presentation was confirmed at the level of molecular biology, biochemistry and the genetics of the familial variety. Improving diagnostic methods, burgeoning scientific literature and consensus conferences where various investigators and clinicians exchange information are instrumental to dispel the myth that the disease is rare. We do not have reliable (population based) counts, but a conservative estimate would be 12% of the dementias, more than a million sufferers in the US alone.[1]

---

1 For the evolution and the history of the disease, and the detailed biography of Arnold Pick and a complete set of references, refer to the book entitled, "Pick's disease and Pick complex," A. Kertesz and D.G. Munoz (editors), published by Wiley-Liss, 1998.

Two

The Banana Lady (Food Fads)

THE PHONE RANG again in the small parish office and Henry knew who was calling before he answered. He lost count, but Dawn had called already several times that morning to make sure he bought milk and bananas on his way home. He gazed at the phone in desperation, considered disconnecting it, but took a deep breath and picked up the receiver.

Dawn, the minister's wife, was competent, socially skilled, musically gifted and working as a receptionist before her illness. She had played an important role in her husband's parish, even entertained the Queen on one of her visits to Canada. She was in her late fifties when she began behaving strangely. She would stand at the edge of a gathering, not talking to people. During other church events, she disappeared upstairs to play the piano. She stopped entertaining and organizing various parish functions and one day, she returned home from work an hour early without explanation. She spent a lot of time in bed, complained of buzzing in her head and insomnia and cried when listening to Christmas carols in a strange display of emotional "incontinence". Her family doctor interpreted her symptoms as depression, but she was not sad and she did not improve on various antidepressants. When she began repeating stories tediously, her family thought there was something wrong with her memory, and this eventually led to a neurological consultation two years after the onset of her symptoms.

By the time she came to the clinic, she had developed another set of strange, disinhibited behaviours. Totally out of character, she greeted her husband with a sexually provocative embrace, and discussed her sex life with strangers. Impulsively she danced the polka in the house. She would get up in the middle of the night and go out on to the street for exercise to help her sleep. As part of her preoccupation with insomnia she began drinking "nightcaps," mainly Scotch. Henry had to hide the bottle from her. When her family doctor suggested she have hot milk and a banana instead of liquor to promote sleep, she began eating 5-6 bananas at a time. Later claiming other foods upset her stomach, she went on a diet of three or four liters of milk and several bunches of bananas a day. She called Henry several times a day at the parish office to make sure there would be enough milk and bananas for her. He restricted her milk intake at night, because of a new problem: bedwetting, but she took to knocking on neighbours' doors to borrow milk or to use their washroom as she roamed the streets.

Initially she needed reminders to do cooking, cleaning, and vacuuming and eventually she stopped doing household chores altogether. Although she had been a cultured woman, she began to watch old Tarzan movies and would surf the channels aimlessly when her husband wanted to watch the news. She returned to topics repeatedly and her songs played on the piano were always the same ones. She misunderstood conversations, and appeared to be very concrete about what she heard. Her youngest son, for instance, made a joke about the girl's hockey team he was coaching, something to the effect: "these girls are so good, they should be playing with boys" and she started worrying about him sleeping with a lot of women.

When I first met Dawn, she was pleasant, talkative, and well oriented, not at all "demented". Her speech was somewhat rambling, tangential, and cheerfully irrelevant. To some, she may have appeared manic, but she also had an air of indifference and lack of insight. The neuropsychologist noted repetitiveness and difficulty concentrating, but her intelligence and immediate memory were surprisingly normal. She did well on the traditional "frontal lobe" tests, with the exception of trail-making, or connecting numbers and letters in an alternating sequence, which requires attention and concentration. Some of her responses appeared slapdash, impulsive, or possibly related to lack of motivation.

Her illness progressed even though some of her roaming and excessive milk and banana intake were incompletely controlled on a medication called Trazodone.[2] New symptoms kept appearing, such as her frequent, compulsive use of the bathroom for which no other medical explanation,

---

2   An antidepressant found to improve some symptoms of FTD. See discussion later on serotonin and treatment.

such as infection or other disease in the urinary tract was found. She became irritable and argumentative when her milk intake was restricted. In addition to her social withdrawal and disinhibition, she neglected her appearance and her family. She would not get dressed in the morning and wore a sweat suit all day long. Initially, she would make lunch for her husband, but eventually they ate only T.V. dinners. She enjoyed going for car rides and liked speed. She would urge Henry to speed across intersections, even though the light was changing.

On a return visit a year later, her restless and distractible behaviour was very evident and disruptive. She got up several times during the interview, walked around the examining room, picked up pictures, books, and touched many other objects. Her speech was less spontaneous and her answers were brief, superficial and glib. She often appeared to be chewing and while she was sitting, moved her body up and down in a stereotypic fashion, like "posting" on horseback.

Eventually, Henry retired to care for her, and carried on valiantly for several more years with the help of homecare workers. He took her bizarre behaviour with equanimity and his sense of humor and selfless, giving personality, combined with his training and experience in ministering to others helped him survive the ordeal. During this time, she developed a craving for chocolate and ate sugar by the spoonful. She would stuff food into her mouth, pocketing it in her cheeks, not swallowing between bites. Her speech decreased and finally she became mute and immobile, not showing any expression or emotion. Eventually she required total nursing care and she was admitted to a nursing home and died after nine years of illness. I saw her husband again a few years later and was pleased to hear he resumed a ministry in the northern community where they moved to in the last few years. He seemed to be the same bright, witty and kind man with a new life.

Her family was interested and agreed to a post-mortem examination of the brain. The findings were quite specific for what is now becoming recognized as the commonest variety of FTD/Pick complex. Atrophy (shrinkage) of the frontal and temporal regions with microscopic deposits or inclusions of degraded protein were found in the nerve cells, similar in location to Pick bodies in Pick's disease but staining like the inclusions in motor neuron disease (MND)[3] (find out more about staining tissues, or histochemistry, an important method in defining disease, in the "Lost and found" chapter). When she was still alive, the typical bilateral frontal and temporal atrophy that gives the disease its anatomic name was seen on computerized tomography (CT), magnetic resonance imaging (MRI) and isotope scans, although her neuroimaging was initially read as age-related change by the radiologist (Fig. 1). (To be fair, in some other instances it is the radiologist who suggests the diagnosis of Pick's disease or FTD in the brain imaging reports).

The story of Dawn is typical of the behavioural presentation of Pick's disease, or frontotemporal degeneration, from the beginning to the end. One of her most remarkable symptoms, suggesting the title, was her food compulsion with certain food preferences, a feature so common that it is considered diagnostic. The obsessive insistence on certain foods, such as

---

3   Known as Lou Gehrig's disease in America after the ballplayer who came down with this progressive wasting of the motor system. It affects strength, swallowing, and speech, but recent studies support that association with FTD is much more common than thought even a few yeas ago.

sweets, bananas, and varieties of spicy "junk food" is the most typical but it can be chicken, fast foods, sauces, Chinese food, and at times, alcohol. Most often other explanations for the craving of sweets such as diabetes are excluded, and the extent of it is clearly more than the "sweet tooth" some of us retain from childhood. Overeating is considered at times a sign of depression, but in FTD/Pick's it has a bizarre, obsessive quality to it. It resembles to some extent "Pica" (originally dirt eating), the peculiar craving of certain foods during pregnancy in some individuals. It can be also seen in autism, when autistic children crave sweet and spicy foods and will refuse to eat anything else. FTD patients share other features with autism and this will be discussed later in the book.

The preference for bananas and certain cookies or types of chips and crackers can be extreme, to the exclusion of other foods in FTD/Pick's. Some buy and consume candies by the bagful, at times finishing all of it in one sitting, qualifying for the label of gluttony. I have dozens of patients who were "addicted" to large quantities of bananas, the lady of our title being one of them. Apparently bananas contain large amounts of the amino acid tryptophane, a precursor of serotonin and it is believed that the deficiency of serotonin in the brain of these individuals is the basis of craving of bananas and other sweets that may serve as chemical stimulants for replenishing the missing neurotransmitters. Although glucose increases serotonin, the neurotransmitter regulating mood and activity in animals, this is only assumed in humans, and the reason for the calming and mood-elevating effects of sugar is not known exactly. The presumed serotonin deficiency also provides a rationale for the use of the serotonin boosting antidepressants (also known as selective serotonin reuptake inhibitors – SSRIs) in this illness with variable success and some improvement of symptoms (Swartz, et al. 1997). A word of caution is necessary concerning the side effects of these frequently used drugs. They are rarely severe, but they should be prescribed and withdrawn only by those fully familiar with them. More will be said about serotonin and its relationship to other behaviours in the next chapter.

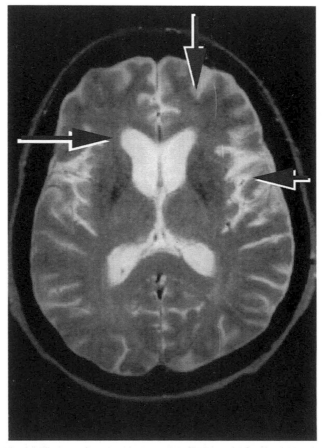

Fig. 1: MRI shows frontal and temporal shrinkage on both sides (arrows).
The dark is brain, white is fluid. Frontal is top. Horizontal slice.

The following quotes are from caregivers who told me about the preoccupation with and craving for sweets and certain other types of food repeatedly. They provide not only the variety (and the lack of variation for each individual, called stereotypy), but also the tone and the intensity of these behaviours that distinguish them from the ordinary food preferences most of us have:

...Developed a sweet tooth, ...craves sweets, coconut cream pies, has started smoking again...has no appetite for anything but pies and sweets...craves ice cream, fruit juice, chicken... developed a craving for sugar, eats a lot of sweets, desserts are her main meal...orders plum sauce with everything, drinks a lot of tea with huge amounts of sugar...always chews gum, has a lot of candy, is obsessed with coffee cake, honey, maple syrup...likes to eat junk food, crackers, cereal, butter tarts, popcorn... eats sugar by the spoonfuls... lives on pop and chips, drinks a lot of beer...drinks wine compulsively, even in the morning, since he bought a book on wine...always wants chocolate and Doritos... preoccupied with eggs, grapefruit and turkey... likes a lot of doughnuts and oatmeal raisin cookies, drinks a lot of juice... wants to have Chinese food all the time, ...craves cinnamon buns and coffee...will eat a whole tub of ice cream for breakfast, craves candy...always buys fig Newtons and bananas...craves chicken sandwiches and French fries...eats excessive amounts of apples, bananas, and chocolate bars...craves oatmeal raisin cookies, always orders chicken at a restaurant...cooks chicken with mushrooms every day...eats raisins soaked in gin 9 times a day...developed a sweet tooth, eats candy, jam, chocolate, and oranges...craves chicken wings...only eats cookies, raisins, and candy, likes dessert, wants to chew gum all the time...goes to

Tim Hortons (doughnut shop) daily...likes chocolate bars, does not know when to stop...wants Lays potato chips every day... diminished food intake except for sweets...loves cookies, drinks a lot of wine...buys sweet drinks, craves chocolate and ice cream... will eat four desserts after a meal...ate a whole cake in two days, eats several bunch of bananas a day...hoards candies...wants to go to Swiss Chalet (a chicken restaurant) all the time.

Dawn had a host of other behaviour and personality changes that prompted her family and friends to say she was not the person they knew before! This dramatic loss of personality was first described in a case report in the middle of the 19th century by a Vermont physician, John Harlow, that concerned a remarkable accident that by itself was worth chronicling. Phineas Gage was a conscientious, reliable railway construction foreman who was neat in his personal habits and observant of social decorum until a long iron rod, used to tap gunpowder for blasting, was blown through his left orbit and frontal lobes. Although he survived the accident without any paralysis, his personality changed remarkably. He became irresponsible, irreverent, childish, and socially inappropriate and as Harlow described it in the paper, "Gage was no Gage anymore." Dawn, like most others in this book, underwent this strange transformation characterized by social inappropriateness, changes in her habits, way of dressing, concrete thinking, childishness, obsessive routines and food fads, coupled with a strange indifference and stubbornness. She changed like Dr. Jekyll to Mr. Hyde, a transformation that matches anything science fiction can devise.

Three

Pickwickian Portions (Gluttony)

D ICK WAS PERSUADED to come to the clinic under false pretenses. His wife told him he needed to be examined for his itchy skin rash. He denied that anything else was wrong and was angry when some of his behaviour was questioned. The referral note suggested he may have Alzheimer's disease. When he was asked what he thought his trouble was, he said he was nervous and scratched himself because of his hives, which was all true, but it was far from the whole story. He reminded me of the "fat boy" from Dickens' Pickwick Papers because of his size, and British (I was told south London) accent. Karen, his wife, became increasingly concerned about his weight and his refusal to take medication for his hypertension. She mentioned his personality change to the family doctor when it became obvious and he was referred to the neurology clinic.

When interviewed alone, Karen recounted a grim tale of Dick beginning to act silly about five years earlier, in his mid-fifties. He just did not know when to stop with his joking and childish teasing. He became rude, loud, and obnoxious, telling his teenage daughters they were ugly or stupid; as a result, they did not want to be around him anymore. His jokes were coarse and he would use four-letter words frequently. His sexual appetite increased to the extent that Karen asked for some medication to control it.

Although he had been an immaculate dresser, he began neglecting his personal hygiene and wore old and dirty clothes. He had to be reminded to take a shower. One day he urinated in a beer glass when the bathroom was only five feet away. Nasty and hurtful remarks dried up their socializing and he had no interest in his friends or entertaining people. Furthermore, he stopped doing anything around the house on his own. When he was asked, he would tell the family they were interfering with his time and he wanted to be left alone. When he occasionally carried out some chores, he made dangerous mistakes such as neglecting to close the propane valves and filling their trailer with gas.

Overeating caused him to top 300 lbs. when he was seen. He literally ate everything in sight, not only what he was served, but also what others left on the table. Half an hour later he would ask for food again. He regularly spent $20 on snacks such as Doritos and chocolate, and ate the lot in one sitting. He would hide food under the sofa and would deny this when confronted. His table manners deteriorated; he would help himself first, starting to eat before everyone else. Later, he demanded that dinner should be served to him in his chair in the living room. He developed accidents with his bladder. It seemed to Karen that he could not be bothered to get up to the washroom.

All day he would do word search games, or watch television. Some of what he watched, he took quite literally. For instance, he insisted he would marry Xena, the "warrior princess," and watched all her shows, but when he was told Xena would not put up with his behaviour he let it go. He would often just sit and make childish noises like playing with cars, "vroom, vroom." When grocery shopping, he would push the cart very fast and would take a can from the cart and throw it at his wife to catch. He would fill out all contest and trial forms that came in the mail and send them away; consequently, Karen received invoices for $380 for books, magazines, videos and an $800 air-walker. He would call 1-800 numbers, psychic lines, and 1-900 numbers for telephone pornography, although he was not interested in real sex anymore. Karen tried to reason with him, but he said, "I can do what I want!"

Three weeks prior to being seen, he chased his daughter's boyfriend out of the house with a hammer and when he was asked what he was doing, he said he was "just kidding." The young people thought he was quite serious and that he was going to use the hammer. His eldest daughter was getting married and when she was saying her vows, "I do," he yelled "No" several times and then laughed. When the groom said he promised to love and cherish her, Dick said, "He's lying. I know he is lying." He bruised his wife after grabbing her for attention to add injury to insult. Karen felt like sinking into the ground; fortunately, most of the wedding guests had heard by then about the changes in Dick and were not too surprised, but some of them experienced his behaviour for the first time.

The family history was ominous, as his mother apparently died at the age of 64 with the diagnosis of "Alzheimer's
disease," but also had a personality change and received
electroshock therapy. She probably had FTD/Pick's disease, but autopsy was not done. His sister died in her early
40s with the diagnosis of a manic depressive illness. One
of his brothers died at the age of 64 from a massive coro-
nary but he lived by himself and had been affected with
odd behaviour; apparently, he had molested a child. His
younger brother, age 41, was still working, but had had
some psychiatric treatment. He became angry with the
mayor so he took a key to the mayor's brand new car and
scratched it and then he told everybody, as he seemed to
think it was very funny. Subsequently he went to jail. The
siblings may also have had FTD/Pick's disease, but two of
them died without autopsy and the living one could not
be reached for verification.

Dick was a large, morbidly obese man on examination
with apoplectic reddish face, swollen discoloured legs
and ankles, with an oozing, excoriated skin rash, worsened by uncontrolled scratching and poor circulation.
After some attention to his rash, he cooperated enough
for us to find his memory surprisingly good; he was oriented and was able to tell me about recent news and
remembered quite a few details about the "peppergate"
affair (a current news item at that time), when reminded.
The Mini Mental State Examination (MMSE)[4] score was a
borderline 27/30, but he refused to have detailed neuropsychological assessment until a year later when his

---

4 The MMSE is a brief screening test of cognition used to screen for dementia. Common cut off
score is 26, above which is a range considered mild cognitive impairment (MCI), or normal. FTD
patients often have normal MMSE even several years into their illness.

card sorting and trail-making tests (of "frontal, executive function") were still within normal limits. Karen, as one would suspect from the history, endorsed many items on the Frontal Behavioral Inventory.[5] Single Photon Emission Computerized Tomography (SPECT)[6] scan showed bilateral temporal impairment particularly on the right side.

He was treated with Trazodone and he improved somewhat on the medication. He was less angry, but as he became more placid he also became practically immobile, unwilling to go anywhere or do anything. It was impossible to get him back for repeated testing. He died at home of a heart attack, three years after he was first seen and approximately eight years after the onset of his illness. Postmortem examination confirmed the diagnosis of Pick complex, but the histology did not detect any inclusions (this seems to occur in the minority of cases and it was labeled "dementia lacking distinctive histology").

Food fads, obsessive food preferences, and gluttony are distinct behaviours of FTD/Pick's disease. These symptoms are not always present, neither are they specific, but when a middle-aged person changes dietary habits in this fashion, in association with other changes of behaviour and personality, all sorts of alarm bells should ring for a diagnosis of FTD/Pick's. In our experience, these behaviours often appear together, but Julie Snowden and her colleagues from Manchester, England suggest they may appear in different groups of patients, those

5 A quantifiable inventory of behaviours, developed at our centre (Kertesz, et al. 1997). A score above 27 is suggestive of FTD and above 30 is confirmatory.
6 Single Photon Emission Computerized Tomography (SPECT) uses isotopes and measures cerebral blood flow, which reflects brain functioning in addition to structural changes on MRI (Magnetic Resonance Imaging). The images are not as clear, but some investigators believe the changes are earlier than on MRI. PET scan has better resolution, but it is expensive and not easily available.

with more left temporal shrinkage having food fads and those
with right sided atrophy having more gluttony (Snowden,
Bathgate, et al. 2001). Dick's neuroimaging, in fact, appears
to confirm this prediction.

Gluttony generally means the indiscriminate eating of larger
quantities than one needs. It could, of course, include taking
that extra helping of a favourite food which most of us indulge
in at one time or another. The ancients considered it one of
the seven deadly sins, but alas, it remained prevalent throughout the ages. From the bible to classical art (e.g. Hyeronymus
Bosch in the Prado museum) to modern crime and comedy
in films, these cardinal sins are recurrent themes. Gluttony is
the 6th circle in Dante's purgatory, next to the top. The neu-
ropsychiatrist Zoltan Janka, among others, made a scholarly
review of the connections between the behaviours of the seven
deadly sins and serotonin deficiency in the brain. Serotonin
is an important neurotransmitter regulating emotions and
behaviour. Serotonin deficiency has been linked to depression,
obsessive compulsive disorders, aggression and eating disorders and medications that increase brain serotonin (SSRI type
antidepressants) are used to treat these conditions.

The Pickwickian syndrome in medicine refers to the respi-
ratory and sleep disturbance associated with obesity. Dickens
immortalized the "fat boy" in his "Pickwick Papers," who
spends his life in an easy chair, often asleep. Obese individuals
with daytime sleepiness often snore heavily and have intermit-
tant cessation of breathing called sleep apnea[7] during the night.
This is considered to produce a lack of oxygen to the brain and
it can be another cause of cognitive impairment, mostly loss of

---

7   Prolonged (more than 10 seconds) pause in breathing, a rather frightening occurrence to the
partner, who is often awake because of the loud snoring.

short-term memory and inattentiveness, but not the behaviour and language disturbance of FTD/Pick's disease. Although Dick was affected by morbid obesity, and he spent most of his later life in an easy chair, his behaviour was related to fronto-temporal degeneration and not attributable to sleep apnea.

Caregivers of FTD patients often remark not only on over-eating or food fads, but also on eating too fast and losing table manners. Their charges help themselves to food before every-one else and keep stuffing themselves until all food is gone. There may not be an obvious increase in reported hunger with the excessive eating, which seems more of a compulsion than a physiological need. When there is no food served, the patient may forget all about eating. Some other individuals watch the clock to see if it is time for a meal, and one patient would set the clock ahead as she was so impatient to get to her favourite restaurant.

Often associated with gluttony are eating faster, wolfing food down, pocketing of food in the mouth without swallowing and eating with fingers instead of utensils. Cecile Marczinski, a psychologist in our unit, recounted an episode: "The patient, who came for neuropsychological testing, became distracted by a lunch item on the shelf. Eyeing the packet of applesauce with a look of eagerness, he said: "I cannot continue this, my head hurts from hunger". When he was offered the snack, the eating of it was impressive in speed, it was like watching a fast forward movie…no time to breath…gobbling it with such an urgency as if he had not eaten in days".

Choking on food tends to occur later in the illness, related partly to eating too fast, partly to food pocketing in the mouth and eventually due to the deterioration of the neural regula-tion of swallowing mechanisms, a frequent terminal event. In the absence of paralysis of the swallowing muscles, it seems to be related to the loss of frontal control of swallowing. In cases associated with motor neuron disease (MND), difficulty swallowing occurs earlier in the course of the disease, as the muscles of the throat become involved, shortening its duration to 2-3 years instead of the average 8-10 years from onset.

Gluttony and sweet craving often result in weight increase, but because it is not always associated with increased hunger in FTD, it might be controlled by less frequent meals and by decreasing the portion served. These individuals may not be that hungry, but eating is a compulsion once food is in front of them. The associated deterioration of social conventions at mealtime is troublesome and embarrassing, and often precludes outings to a restaurant or social gatherings. The compulsive consumption might extend from sweet drinks to alcohol and if this is viewed out of context, the mistaken diagnosis of alcoholism may be made. Some of this behaviour may be considered under the umbrella of the general loss of social conduct or disinhibition, rather than hyperorality, as defined and discussed below and it is an example of the overlap between the terms and explanations for these behaviours. The following quotes from the caregivers in my practice illustrate gluttony:

>...Sits down, loads her plate and starts eating before everybody else ...eats quickly...would drink alcohol excessively if allowed, loves to eat everything in general...puts more food on her plate, eats more than usual...takes other people's food...puts everything in her mouth...started over-eating, always seems to be hungry...keeps food in his mouth like a chipmunk, needs verbal reminders to swallow...wolfs his meal down...gobbles food...eats five chocolate bars in one sitting...can hardly wait

until dinner comes, eats food from other people's plates when he is done with his own...eats a lot quicker...consumes large amounts of food...constantly reaches for food and drinks everything in sight...puts too much food in his mouth, drools...finishes the whole chocolate cake left in the fridge...eats everything, does not know when to stop...has an excessive appetite...pushes food in her mouth to the point of choking on it..., eats excessively everything that is in front of him, drinks as much wine as he can...compulsive eating...stuffs herself as if she were starving...finishes meals much more quickly than others... practically inhales food... eats very quickly, will eat almost two meals at each sitting... shoves food in his mouth ...eats snack food right after a big meal...puts everything in his mouth...picks at other people's food...bites into anyone or anything...puts foreign objects in her mouth...puts her fingers in her mouth a lot.... stuffs food in her cheeks without swallowing.

A link has been made between gluttony, food fads, and later on, the indiscriminate placing of all sorts of objects in the mouth, under the overall label of hyperorality. In the mid-thirties a physiologist, Heinrich Kluver, and a neurosurgeon, Paul Bucy, in Chicago, carried out a series of surgical procedures on monkeys in order to observe the effects of temporal lobectomies for the treatment of epilepsy. These now famous experiments resulted in peculiar behaviours in these animals and similar symptoms in humans are often remembered as the Kluver-Bucy syndrome. The animals, after recovering from bilateral removal of their temporal lobes, were not impaired physically, but exhibited hyperactive, hypersexual, and hyperoral behaviours. They explored everything, fondling objects, including snakes placed in their cages, even putting them in their mouth. This would never have occurred prior to surgery, since all primates, monkeys, and apes, including humans, are terrified of reptiles.

This behaviour was called "oral tendencies" by Kluver and Bucy and had several interpretations. One was focused on their inability to recognize objects, called visual agnosia. This is not blindness, or a deficit of perception, but a lack of recognition of the nature and the meaning of the objects. Agnosia (Greek for not knowing, or not recognizing) will be discussed later in another context of semantic impairment, or loss of meaning in FTD/Pick's. In later stages of FTD/Pick's disease, hyperorality becomes indiscriminate, extending to inedible objects. Occasionally, the most incomprehensible of all behaviours, coprophagia (the eating of feces) appears, probably related to the failure to recognize what the substance is. Fortunately, this is uncommon and occurs in later stage, institutionalized patients. Others interpreted hyperorality as regression to an infantile state of oral exploration of the environment. The Kluver-Bucy type of hyperorality in humans is also associated with excessive touching and manipulating of objects when individuals explore everything in their environment. Our next patient is described as an example of this behaviour.

Four

Keeping in Touch
(Utilization Behaviour)

W HAT MAKES THE NEXT STORY UNIQUE, is that it is based on the detailed, typewritten, notes of a caregiver with a literary bent, providing an extra flavour to the description of the behavioural presentation of FTD/Pick's disease. The title refers to the phenomenon of compulsive touching and use of objects, frequently observed in FTD/Pick's. He had developed a host of other problems, but this was particularly striking because of the extent and manner in which he began using every container and receptacle in the house. His "utilization behaviour", although extreme, was only one aspect of the multifaceted symptoms of FTD/Pick's syndrome. It is also a story of a recent marriage, a promise of a new life gone inexplicably awry, and a new wife learning to cope and to endure an extraordinary burden she had not bargained for.

Keith was a bachelor farmer and a mechanic. His work-
shop and tool collection was larger than some in commer-
cial garages. When he met Debbie, a single mother of a
handicapped son, they thought they were made for each
other. Curiously, years before they met, a fortuneteller told
Debbie, by then alone, ..." later in your life you are going
to have another child"... About a year after Keith married at
the age of 43 his behaviour took a strange turn. Debbie was
struck by his lack of ambition. Projects did not get finished
and he sold his animals and cut down his machinery repair
business. They rented the farm out, because he lost interest in it. His disinterest extended to all aspects of life; he
did not want to call his friends or make any decisions.

Problems really came to a head when they went to Florida.
Before they went on the trip he cashed in an investment,
which was in poor judgment, because they did not need
the cash. He became agitated and anxious about the whole
process of renting a car and he wanted to take it back and
stay at the airport for a week. He was preoccupied about
running out of money and he would not participate in any
of the activities Debbie suggested, such as swimming or
a boat ride, but they did take on an all day cruise to the
Bahamas on a casino boat. During the voyage he repeatedly asked the ship's staff what time it was in the Bahamas.
In the dining room he insisted on having a fried egg sandwich. Bananas, pecan and apple pie became a recurring
staple. He kept buying maps of Florida, often the same
ones, but never looked at them. His wife had to navigate as
he refused to let her drive. The rental car acquired a yellow
paint streak on the last day, but he told the agency it had
been there when they picked it up. When they came home

he insisted on going back to the plane for his luggage, even though it was checked in and he was supposed to receive it in the baggage area. After a cab ride he claimed it only cost 35 cents and when his wife asked him if he meant $35.00 he became adamant that the guy only asked for 35 cents. His fibbing, stubbornness and argumentativeness were definite changes in personality from the Keith Debbie had known.

Later, Debbie also noticed a decline in personal hygiene. Keith needed prompting about showers and not to hang his dirty clothes back in the closet. He wore a t-shirt hanging out from under his jacket, but his wife excused this initially as he was never much of a dresser on the farm. He began to seek permission to do everything, not being able to decide, "Should I have my bath now or should I have it later?" He kept asking what day it was and similar questions again and again. Although he was a licenced mechanic, he did not realize or did not seem to care that their car was falling apart, the heater did not work, there were holes in the exhaust and fumes were entering the car. He could not install a baseboard heater in the bathroom, but refused to call an electrician.

At family gatherings he was withdrawn, would look through an album or a book compulsively rather than make conversation, and he would not talk to his wife's handicapped son who lived with them even though he had been kind and attentive to him in the past. He started doing large jigsaw puzzles, over 100 pieces. He leafed through books, but could not persist reading them, or to watch a T.V. show to the end. He would lie on the couch all day, if his wife let him. He did not bother answering the phone or going to the door and did not recognize a neighbour who came to visit. He would find humour in things Debbie did not think were funny, such as decrepit barns and strange looking mailboxes, making jokes that these should be their next place. He refused to make a dental appointment or go to his doctor for a check-up. Eventually the family doctor saw him and diagnosed Alzheimer's disease, but neuroimaging suggested frontotemporal atrophy and he was referred for a neurological assessment.

In my office he behaves childishly with silly gestures, points his finger at me like a gun and clicks his tongue, imitating a shot. He raises his eyebrows and has a frequent silly laugh and an incongruous, unwarranted, fatuous smile. In the waiting room he was seen pulling the zipper of his fly up and down repetitively. He is oriented, but pays little attention to memory items and he does not register or recall anything from a story. He does poorly on tests of complex executive function requiring attention, shifting concepts such as card sorting, trail-making, and finding words in a category. He gets up and gathers the cards and other testing material when he wants to stop. He volunteers nothing but when he is asked, he talks in full sentences. His score on the Frontal Behavioural Inventory is 40, which is well above the diagnostic cut off score of 30 for FTD. His MRI shows bilateral frontotemporal atrophy.

When he came back a year later, Debbie provided further disturbing details. He was restless and wanted to go out and drive, but his licence was revoked so she ended up driving him around up to 100 miles a day. He loved roaming the malls and thrived on visual stimulation. He walked restlessly around stores, but never bought anything. He repeatedly asked his wife when she was going to pick him up at the front door and insisted she park the car as close to the mall entrance as possible. He watched the clock obsessively, and as he kept checking his watch he asked everybody to coordinate their watches. At a restaurant he made beeping noises like the Three Stooges. Before he started to eat, he mixed his food together and poured his drink into his food. He developed a sweet tooth, eating several cookies before sandwiches during lunch and he went to Tim Horton's[8] regularly for oatmeal-raisin cookies and doughnuts. He did not like waiting in line and would cut right in. Somebody told him off and his wife had to apologize. Still, he insisted going there three or four times a day. He went to washrooms frequently and Debbie was not sure whether or not he needed to, or if this had just become a new habit. He loved bananas, eating five or six a day, and stuffed too much food into his mouth.

Hoarding food in a night table or cupboard, including packages of cookies, cans of pop and bottles of juice, became routine. He also bought items repetitively, and excessively, toothpaste for a while and then lightbulbs, well after his wife told him they did not need any more. When Debbie tried to discuss some of these behaviours he would not admit that there was anything wrong. He later became very clingy, dependent on her, and never left her alone. When she had to leave him, he would become anxious, agitated, and paced the floor. For this reason, she stopped taking him to the day care program. He became more and more childlike and had a temper when he was told he could not do something. He shot at police cars with his fingers, also at birds flying in the air, at the source of music and whenever he saw messy bins or

---

8   A Canadian chain of doughnut shops.

messy shelves. He would dance to the music at a department store, oblivious to anyone watching him. He flipped through magazines in the stores and found humour in all sorts of pictures, laughing at things not obviously funny. He repeated the word "Texas" enthusiastically and laughed about it. "Texas" was an answer to many of her questions to him.

He fussed about car windows, the trunk of their car, rearranged the silverware drawer, cursing when he found the spoons out of alignment. He liked folding and rearranging laundry. He frequently touched articles in stores and had a habitual way of stooping to look more closely at things he found interesting. When he went in a store he rearranged merchandise on the shelves or straightened grocery carts. Debbie had to keep him out of grocery stores, because he touched the food. In the bank he would rearrange the pamphlets at each wicket, whether there were customers or not. He often took his wallet out and thumbed through his money. He kept dumping ashes in cans and garbage bins, but never emptied anything. His most disturbing "utilization" behaviour was using rubber boots, boxes, or whatever containers he could find, to urinate into. Debbie cleaned the basement of anything he could use to discourage this behaviour, but then he continued piddling into heat registers on the floor, and in the garden. He denied this childishly when he was confronted with it. He did not do it on the street or in the mall, for which Debbie was grateful.

Neuropsychological testing was a frustrating experience as he gave impulsively inaccurate and perseverative answers. For instance, he knew the date but in response to asking what the year was he said, "the 24th," which was the date. His language was essentially intact, but he would not read or cooperate with other requests. The frontal assessment battery showed a low score[9]. He could not provide similarities and kept perseverating with the word "excellent" when asked what two objects were alike. He refused to find words in a category. His motor sequencing of Luria's[10] "fist-edge-palm" test, imitating the examiner, was poor and he could not do tasks with alternating directions. Many of his cognitive problems were related to his impulsivity, perseveration and lack of motivation.

He was started on Trazodone to control some of the behavioural problems such as the irritability, the compulsive behaviour and roaming. Unfortunately, he developed a rash from it. Other serotoninergic medications and cholinesterase inhibitors helpful in Alzheimer's disease did not seem to help him. He has since developed urinary and fecal incontinence and lately he does not seem to recognize feces, licking it off his fingers. He does not name objects or know what to do with them most of the time, but curiously he can still dress himself and distinguish a convertible or a truck from a choice of four, and chooses Africa instead of farm when seeing a picture of a giraffe. He is echolalic (repeats occasionally sentences uttered by others) but his speech output is restricted to perseverating with stock phrases: "...I just did it when I went between Georgetown and Brampton"... Most follow-up efforts were spent to counsel his wife, who continues to take care of this childish, stubborn, socially and personally deteriorated man in quiet desperation, asking, "What is next?" She has adapted remarkably, but is beginning to lose sleep in the effort to keep him clean at night.

---

9 This is a brief practical examination of executive functions from a French-US collaboration led by Dubois et al.

10 Luria was a Russian neuropsychologist famous for his analytical, yet practical methods of examining brain injured individuals and frontal lobe function.

Compulsive stereotypic routines, clock watching, perseverations, restless roaming, and compulsive touching
are often overlapping and occur simultaneously with other
changes in personality. Touching everything creates problems in shops, restaurants, making outings less desirable and
eventually impossible. More will be said about this later in
conjunction with hoarding and shoplifting.

The phenomenon of patients going around a room, uninvit-
edly examining, and using objects, has attracted the attention
of clinicians and investigators in various forms of frontal lobe
injury. In the case of Keith, this took unpleasant and disturbing
forms such as rearranging shelves in a supermarket and urinating in any available container. This overall behaviour is also
named "environmental dependency" because patients behave as
if they were dependent on exploring their environment for continuing existence, very similar to an infant or a toddler exploring
his or her new world, or the Kluver- Bucy monkeys touching
and putting everything in their mouth. This, of course, overlaps
with hyperorality, discussed previously.

The French neurologist, Francois Lhermitte, examining
patients with frontal lobe injury, used the term "utilization
behaviour". His method of testing was to put utensils or writing implements in front of the patients to see if they would
use them without being asked (normal individuals usually
would not). This is a subtler phenomenon than the spontaneous, continuous touching and grabbing of some of the more
advanced patients. In later stages of FTD/Pick's, a forced
grasp reflex may develop when the patient has trouble releas-
ing anything grasped, at times to the extent that the fingers
have to be pried open. Keith's utilization of all sorts of recep-
tacles for urinating may be an extreme and complex form

of utilization behaviour combined with social disinhibition. Dick in the previous chapter also had this in a milder form (urinated in a glass instead of getting up to the bathroom).

Many descriptions of utilization behaviour and environmental dependency were in cases of head injuries or brain tumors of the frontal lobes or as the sequel of encephalitis or stroke. However, these are usually dramatic, sudden events (except tumors, which can be slowly growing and insidious), and should not be difficult to differentiate by a skilled specialist. Neuroimaging, preferably with magnetic resonance imaging (MRI), is helpful not only to confirm the shrinkage in the frontotemporal lobes, but also to detect a slowly growing brain tumor or inflammation of the brain that could account for the behavioural change.

Some examples of compulsive touching and utilization as observed by in FTD/Pick patients are listed here:

Reaches out and touches everything...picks her fingers constantly...likes to hold people's hands...scrapes the table with her utensils...picks things up and fiddles with them...attempts to use everything in front of her...would take things in a store if allowed to...constantly rattles and pushes her cutlery...constantly touches everything...picks up something and says "hmm"...picks at things within reach...pats children's heads...picks up and sniffs and smells all food...touches everything in sight...picks up spoon and fork, picks up and puts down pop cans...started playing with her clothes and buttons...she is always touching things...tears up cardboard, brushes everything with her hand, turns the water tap on and off, rubs material...touches items absentmindedly...plays with her purse...reads aloud signs and labels... he was often fidgety, manipulating objects for no reason... touches objects repetitively...

picks at things compulsively...takes out his wallet and plays with money, thumbing banknotes... claps with her hands...picks at her nails...goes up to coworkers and touches them, grabs things out of others' hands...fond of touching certain surfaces, such as corduroy, scratches surfaces of plastic containers... goes around and around an empty plate with a fork...

Keith also had a great number of compulsive routines also called stereotypies, in many ways overlapping with utilization behaviours. Some of these are going to be discussed in more detail and compared to other obsessive-compulsive behaviours in chapter 15. The earliest changes were, however, apathy, disinterest and indifference, documented carefully by Debbie in her lengthy chronicles of her husband's illness. Apathy and disinterest are not specific and are also symptoms of depression and Alzheimer's disease, which are the most common initial misdiagnosis. However, apathy in FTD occurs without the sadness, thoughts of worthlessness or suicidal ideation of depression. Sooner or later restless roaming, as in the case of Keith, compulsions and disinhibition appear, confirming the suspicion that the apathy is not related to depression, but to FTD. Interestingly, the Kluver-Bucy syndrome also included apathy, placidity and compliance, paradoxical as it may seem, associated with the excessive exploratory behaviour in the experimental animals and in the example of Keith. More about apathy, aspontaneity, disengagement, disinterest and their biological and biochemical relationships in chapter 17.

Five

Speechless in Sarnia
(Primary Progressive Aphasia)

B ILL'S STORY DIFFERS enough from the others in this book, that for a while his type of illness was considered a separate entity, even though Arnold Pick clearly described the same language loss in his original papers, in association with the behavioural disorder. However when it occurs in relative isolation, it is often mistaken for a stroke or an emotional disorder or described as a new disease. It was labeled first as Primary Progressive Aphasia (PPA) and relabeled as Progressive Non-fluent Aphasia (PNFA). Careful observation of these patients over the years reveals the relationship to the behavioural and motor varieties of FTD/Pick's. Some degree of language loss is the rule in all varieties, although it may come later in the course of the illness, after the behavioural presentation. This may not get the same attention as in those instances when it comes first (it is primary). There are several varieties, although what is described below seems to be the most common and the most distinct.

Bill was 64 years old and retired from his professional engineering career in the"chemical valley" of Sarnia, Ontario, when he began experiencing word finding difficulties, mixing up words and stuttering. His speech gradually worsened, becoming garbled according to his family and at times difficult to understand. Writing was also affected, particularly forming letters, and this was attributed to weakness of the right hand. He did not seek help for two years mainly because the symptoms were mild and he continued to function well. First he was diagnosed as having had a stroke and was put on Aspirin. He continued to drive a car, took care of the gardening, banking, keeping books, and his memory was still good for remembering appointments and recent events. He made spelling and sometimes grammatical errors in his diary. Because of continuing deterioration he was referred for further investigation.

Four years after onset, at the age of 68, the neurological examination showed a mild tremor of the hands, the right more than the left, but otherwise he appeared physically and psychiatrically normal. He was fully oriented, pleasant and cooperative, but his speech was seriously disturbed, halting and hesitant as he stumbled on initial syllables, frequently repeating, and often distorting them. He had a great deal of difficulty finding words and he produced incomplete sentences or just a single word answer. What speech he had was much segmented; each word was separately emphasized so that the normal fluency and melodic line of the sentence was interrupted. His comprehension was good, except for complex commands. Naming objects was only slightly impaired. He could not whistle, click his tongue, or show how to salute or use a hammer; in technical terms he had significant facial and limb apraxia.[11]

His son documented his decline in extensive, respectful, even loving notes, sometimes quite poignantly: "His vocabulary diminished further and he rarely initiated conversation, but he still read a great deal and appeared to fully comprehend what he was reading. He continued driving, gardening, advising his family financially, and he still appeared to have an oar for music, responding by humming or attempting to sing along with the band. At 70 he gave up driving voluntarily but remained socially active, going out with friends regularly." A year later his vocabulary was reduced to "yah, yah" and "no, no." His comprehension diminished and he had some difficulty responding to verbal commands. He was still living at home, walked about and socialized with the family, but he showed increasing difficulty caring for himself and his wife assisted him with grooming. At this time he was losing interest in financial matters.

On the second neurological assessment, eight years after the onset, he was mute and severely apractic. He had a rapid tremor, stiffness and immobility of the right hand and trouble turning and shifting position (See Chapter 7 for a more detailed description of this movement disorder, also called corticobasal degeneration). He communicated by pointing at times, but this was inconsistent. He was unable to write or draw. He could not name objects and he licked them when they were put in his hands for demonstrating object use. This

---

11 Apraxia is a form of severe clumsiness or impairment of complex movement or inability to use implements, not due to weakness or incoordination.

form of hyperorality is reminiscent of the oral behaviours in the Kluver-Bucy experiments and to some extent of the utilization behaviour discussed in the previous chapter.

Nine years after onset, he developed urinary incontinence, a year later bowel incontinence and began falling. Lifting his legs into the bathtub became difficult because of stiffness and a curious motor clumsiness. Nevertheless, he continued to recognize acquaintances, remain thoughtful and loving towards his spouse, have an interest in shopping and in music with excited and positive response to familiar tunes, even getting up to dance at the Legion Hall. He was able to go to Florida for a vacation. Despite his deterioration, a loving family, more than willing to care for him, surrounded him.

He was last seen in our department at the age of 73. He was still saying, "yah, yah" with some degree of emphasis and emotional undertone, but he could not be relied upon to reply to yes and no questions. However, on personal questions his response appeared more enthusiastic for 'yes' than for 'no' in a rather appropriate fashion. His formal test scores were all at a floor level, he had a global, all pervasive aphasia, and he would not even select nonverbal stimuli or put puzzles together. His right hand appeared quite rigid and remained in a position where it was placed. When it was lifted in front of him he spread his fingers like a robot, but he could not use them and the hand appeared "alien" as if it did not belong to him.[12]

Ten years after onset he was admitted to a nursing home because of frequent falls. He was still able to learn the location of his room and communicated his familiarity with these

---

12 Alien hand is a feature of corticobasal degeneration, part of the Pick complex. (see the subsequent discussion in the chapter "alien").

locations by turning into these rooms while walking with assistance. He stayed most of the time confined to a geriatric chair, bending at the waist, unable to look up and died 11 years after the onset of his illness. An autopsy showed Pick's disease with Pick bodies (spherical silver staining inclusions in the neurons). MRI (Fig. 2) showed left central and parietal involvement, the areas responsible for processing language and praxis (gestures, practiced movements).

Ravel, the famous composer of Bolero, developed primary progressive aphasia in his early sixties, which remained undiagnosed. He died prematurely as a result of a surgical exploration of his brain in a desperate attempt to reverse his inexorable loss of musical expression along with his language. He retained comprehension and music appreciation (like Bill) for a long time and complained bitterly that he had all this music in his brain but could not play it or write it down. His illness was documented by the French neurologist, Alajouanine, in a scholarly paper called "Artistic Realization in Aphasia" and in a more recent film, using contemporary clips and posthumous reminiscences by friends, titled "Ravel's Brain." In this avant garde "operatic" documentary the role of the operating surgeon, Vincent Clovis, was sung by an opera singer, to dramatize the events leading to Ravel's death (quite absurdly and unsuccessfully in my opinion, perhaps only matching the experimental nature and the futility of the surgery itself. He died a few weeks after surgery). Alajouanine's article focuses on the parallel nature of language and music loss, and no recognition is made of Pick's disease, partly because autopsy was not permitted. Therefore, the true nature of his illness remains a matter of speculation, but the contemporary documentation of his progress including unilateral left hemispheric atrophy on the pneumoencephalogram[13] is diagnostic of primary progressive aphasia in retrospect.

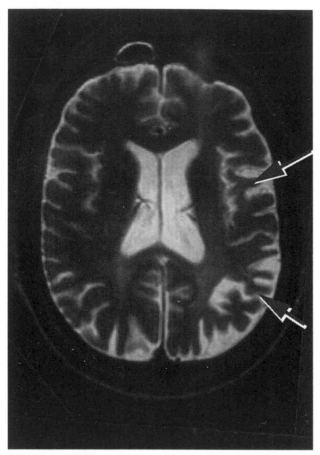

Fig.2: MRI shows left central and parietal shrinkage (language and praxis). Dark is brain. White is fluid. Front is top. Left is on the right side. Aphasia and Apraxia.

---

13 A painful procedure of injecting air into the ventricles, or fluid filled spaces in the brain to provide contrast for x-rays, thankfully replaced by modern neuroimaging of CT and MRI.

Progressive aphasia or loss of language is one of the cardinal features of FTD/Pick's disease. When it is the first symptom to appear, in up to 30-40% of cases, the adjective "primary" is used. Primary progressive aphasia may be seen without cognitive impairment in other domains or personality change for several years, as was the case with Bill. Initially, the aphasia is mild, consisting of word finding difficulty. If it features stuttering, stumbling over words, the term aphemia or verbal apraxia may be used. Bill progressed to a nonfluent aphasia, similar to Broca's aphasia, and later became mute with preservation of a substantial amount of nonverbal cognition.

Paul Broca was a French surgeon and amateur anthropologist who had a patient with speech loss at the time when the uniqueness of speech to human evolution and the human brain was hotly debated by the Paris Anthropological Society. This particular patient was known on the wards of the Salpetrier Hospital in Paris as Tan-tan because his speech was restricted to repetitive stereotypic syllables ... *Tan...tan*. Broca presented the anatomical findings on Tan-tan's brain to the anthropological society in 1861 to support his claim that language was localized in the left hemisphere and launched the extensive study of language localization. Since then patients with similar difficulty of speech characterized by effortful, distorted articulation, agrammatic or telegrammatic (few essential words only) output and well retained comprehension are called Broca's aphasics. A number of PPA patients like Bill go through a phase of resembling Broca's aphasia, but many just have increasing word finding difficulty and simply talk less and less, losing fluency gradually on their way to mutism.

Tremor and rigidity in Bill's right hand were present early, suggesting corticobasal degeneration syndrome (CBDs), the movement disorder of FTD/Pick complex (see the chapter "Alien" for further explanation). Frontal lobe symptoms, hyperorality, severe apraxia and alien hand developed late in his illness. He also had symptoms of progressive supranuclear palsy, which are frequent falls, rigidity, and paralysis of vertical gaze at the end stage of his illness (see also the "Hero of Bolero"). Although Bill had both CBD syndrome in the relatively early to middle stages of his illness and PSP in the end stage, the pathology was classical Pick's disease. Now if this appears to be confusing to a layperson, they may derive a little solace from knowing it has confounded most physicians, especially when they first encounter these changing diagnoses. Those, who do not have the experience or opportunity to follow a sufficient number of these patients, have difficulty understanding the convergence of seemingly different syndromes.

PPA seems to be associated more frequently with CBD and abnormal tau protein positive pathology, while Semantic Aphasia or dementia (see next two chapters) goes with the behavioural variety and tau negative histology, but there is too much overlap to separate these into distinct diseases at this stage of our knowledge. (For an explanation of the role of the tau protein in the disease see the chapter "Lost and Found".) There is much to be learned, but the most productive area of research at this point, the "hottest" if you like, is in the area of molecular biology of the affected proteins.

Several varieties of PPA have been described, but some of this variability probably reflects the stage at which the patient is examined and to a lesser extent a difference in the disease process. Bill, for instance, had only word finding difficulty or "anomia" in the early stages of his illness. Subsequently, stuttering "aphemia" and later loss of speech output characteristic of "nonfluent progressive aphasia" (this is often considered a distinct variety) and finally mutism developed. Many FTD/PPA patients go through these stages and the fluent-nonfluent distinction is arbitrary and difficult to define. Some patients do not stutter or have verbal apraxia, but progressively speak less and less (logopenia). Comprehension remains intact for a relatively long time in contrast to semantic dementia (see chapters on "What is steak?" and "Houdini") where it is lost early in the illness. Although these presentations are different and described under different disease labels, many of us believe they are the same illness, the difference being only whether the more anterior (in cases of PPA or nonfluent progressive aphasia or aphemia) or the more posterior (semantic aphasia or dementia) language areas of the brain are affected first and foremost.

Six

What is Steak?
(Semantic Dementia)

M EMORY HAS BEEN compartmentalized in several ways, such as short term and long term, explicit and implicit (with or without awareness) and semantic memory, which includes our knowledge of concepts, words, names and their meanings, in contrast to episodic memory, which is memory for events, dates, and episodes. It is the episodic, explicit memory that people are mostly concerned about when they visit their doctor or talk to their friends. They also typically complain of losing short term memory, meaning recent memory in contrast to older autobiographical memory, which is typically preserved in aging. This "temporal gradient" is exaggerated in disease such as early Alzheimer's.

Semantic memory on the other hand is hidden, implicit. We take for granted the meaning of words and much of our knowledge about the word. We know food is for eating, water is essential for life and products of elimination are to be cleaned up. We have a huge amount of such knowledge common to everyone from a five-year-old bushman child from the Kalahari to the Queen of England, divergent as it may become with education, experience and culture. Semantic memory has certain properties such as being acquired early in childhood, being over-learned and accessible through multiple modalities, such as vision, hearing, and touch. It is essential to recognize objects, locations, and individuals, and it is instrumental in cognition and language. A cardinal feature of semantic dementia is the loss of meaning for common words with relative preservation of episodic memory for occurrences and episodes and the preservation of conversational speech at least initially. Such a selective loss in Rita in this story left her family and her physicians puzzled and incredulous.

Rita was in her early sixties, when she astonished her husband one day when in reply to his request to have steak for supper she asked: *"What is steak?"* Even before this happened she would become concerned when she forgot the names of flowers and animals. She was referred for forgetfulness with a diagnosis of Alzheimer's disease. It became evident however, that her difficulty finding names was not the same what is ordinary for elderly individuals or early Alzheimer patients, because she also seemed to have lost the meaning of some common words when they came up conversation. In fact, this seemed so bizarre to her husband that he thought she was "putting it on." This did not affect her life substantially at the beginning. She lived on a small farm and she managed her own banking and shopping quite well and her friends and relatives helped her when she was searching for words. Soon, however, she began having trouble cooking because she could not understand labels in the supermarket and did not even recognize the spices or vegetables, when she saw them at home. By the time she was seen, she was having difficulty following conversations and could not understand the newspaper or television programs, even though her own speech remained fluent. She began feeling uneasy at social gatherings and became upset when she could not recall the names of her grandchildren. She was treated with Prozac for depression without any improvement and later she was enrolled in a study of cholinesterase inhibitors for Alzheimer's disease.

Her difficulty with the meaning of common nouns became evident in the fifth or sixth year of her illness. When in the course of testing she was asked to give the name of vehicles in a test of word finding or "word fluency" she would ask:

"What is a vehicle?"

When it was explained to her that it is a method of transportation she would say:

"Oh yes, it is something we drive on but I can't think of any. Another thing that is gone that made a difference to me: the names of places. I used to enjoy television but they spend so much time talking about places that have no meaning to me. However, places close to home such as Kitchener, Cambridge, and Guelph I know." (These place names were altered for the sake of confidentiality.)

In contrast to the loss of semantic memory, her personal or episodic memory was preserved. She remembered when she visited her sister, where they had gone, what they had done and remained oriented in her own environment. She continued to drive and shop with the help of lists. Her spontaneous speech remained fluent, but she made some semantic substitutions such as saying, "catalogue" for "calendar". Seven years after the onset of her illness she was still oriented to time and place, however, when she was asked the name of the province in which we live, she asked:

"What is a province?"

When she was asked again what a steak was she would say,

"I don't know, I can't think what it looks like."

When she was asked how she would cook it anyway she replied,

"I guess steak must be meat",

showing recognition with some verbal-semantic cueing. Nonverbal and non-semantic aspects of her cognition remained surprisingly preserved. For instance she could spell words backwards as spelling requires primarily phonological (the sounds of speech) processing and working memory but not the processing of meaning. Mathematical tasks, such as serial subtractions of 7's from 100 all the way down were done quickly and accurately. Although she copied intersecting pentagons, she could not draw a clock from memory and asked: "What is a clock?" She remembered telephone numbers and continued to be spatially well oriented and drove faultlessly.

On subsequent visits she showed signs of neglecting herself; she was always dressed in the same sweat suit. Her cooking became increasingly restricted to ready-made foods as she lost the meaning of ingredients and seasonings. Repeating words was preserved, even those she did not know the meaning of anymore. When she had to write irregular words she did not know the meaning of, she did it phonetically, for instance, when the word "ache" was dictated she wrote, "ake". Similarly, when it came to reading

irregular words such as 'yacht' she would pronounce them
as if they were regular: "yatcht." She was able to write sentences or repeat them when they were read to her even
though she did not comprehend them[14.]

She had a surprising preservation of colour naming and
she had no trouble matching unknown faces when it came
to a purely visual process of selecting them from multiple
choices, but she could not name familiar or famous faces
requiring meaningful semantic association. Further experiments showed this was not the failure to access names that
Alzheimer patients develop later on in their illness, but a
true loss of meaning in all modalities, even when objects
were presented to her visually, by touch, or smell, or when
she was asked to demonstrate their use. Even though verbal
cues or multiple probes promoted recognition initially, indicating that the semantic associations of each object were
only weakened but not totally absent, subsequently the
items seemed to disappear entirely from her semantic storage. The extensive linguistic and neuropsychological inves-
tigations of Rita became the subject of a scientific paper.[15]

We tried several medications but she continued to dete-
riorate regardless of the treatment she received. Not being
able to recognize most objects around her and not being
able to understand what people said to her became severely
incapacitating. She could not brush her teeth without help
and had no idea what to do with money. She gained weight
as she was eating even when she was full and she developed

---

14 This was known as transcortical sensory aphasia in the neurological literature, because transcortical associations considered essential for processing meaning were impaired, but subcortical
transfer of the heard word to the pronounced one remained intact, enabling the individual to repeat
words without necessarily knowing what they meant.
15 Primary progressive semantic aphasia. Kertesz et al., Journal of the International
Neuropsychological Society 1998;4:388-398.

a liking to everything that had red colour. For instance, she put ketchup on her apple pie. She was still speaking in fluent sentences, but her speech became rather empty and devoid of meaningful nouns. She would say, pointing to cars on the street: *"It is fascinating to see all those things moving around and everything bouncing around"*. Automatic reading without meaning remained preserved. For example, when she was presented with a pack of matches that she could not name and did not know what it was, she would read the label, *"Shopper's Drug Mart, everything you want in a drug store"* with perfectly fluent pronunciation. Subsequently, she became increasingly mute, unable to take care of her basic needs and she was admitted to a nursing home.

Gerald, Rita's husband, was not the only one puzzled by her repeated questioning of the meaning of common words. Most first time observers of this behaviour have trouble fathoming what is happening. The individual affected can carry on a reasonable conversation, while losing the meaning of some words, usually nouns, representing "things". The selective loss of meaning of objects is a striking deficit while there is still preserved conversational speech, phonology, syntax, reading and writing. This loss is parallel with what is commonly known as "fund of knowledge", yet compatible with the retention of episodic memory for personal events and locations known as "autobiographical memory." The pattern is different from progressive aphasics, such as the patient described in "Speechless in Sarnia," who lose speech output (phonology, syntax and access to words), but retain comprehension and understand the meaning of things.

Aphasia or language impairment due to stroke also occurs most often in association with severe problems in articulation, repetition, phonological and syntactic processing and there is a loss of access to words, rather than a loss of meaning. An exception is the so called transcortical sensory aphasia observed after certain strokes affecting the posterior portion of the left hemisphere. These patients in many respects resemble semantic dementia, but the onset is unmistakably sudden and recovery usually follows. Aphasia due to Alzheimer's disease is initially mild and fluent and eventually becomes associated with loss of comprehension at later stages, but the dramatic, early loss of meaning, characteristic of semantic dementia is different. Furthermore, Alzheimer patients lose episodic memory and visuospatial function, which is preserved in semantic dementia or aphasia. This "double dissociation" of cognitive deficits enables the distinction to be made between them.

Patients with semantic dementia initially retain a vocabulary, as well as a certain amount of biographical (personal) and episodic memory pertaining to their daily life. Rita, even though she had difficulty naming, recalling and comprehending common "things", could still use abstract concepts, verbs, verb phrases, and grammatical words with considerable facility. She could talk about her family and her immediate environment and what was happening around her. One could say Rita lived and talked about her world in terms of personal actions, relationships, and her neighborhood environment, yet lacked the meaning of many living and non-living entities, distant locations and non-personal knowledge.

Linguists have compartmentalized language processing to:
1. Phonology, or the knowledge of the rules of pronunciation and perception of the sounds of language. Speakers of any

language acquire the processes of phonology in the first two or three years of their lives, but the rules of phonology can be learned later for other languages as well, even though it becomes more difficult beyond a critical period after puberty. Most of us can not acquire a foreign language without an accent beyond this critical period.

2. Semantics or the systematic knowledge of the meaning of words, symbols and even gestures.

3. Syntax or grammar incorporating the rules of the relationship and shape of words, phrases and sentences, or units of propositional speech, essential to convey accurate meaning.

4. Pragmatics, or the rules of maintaining the give and take of conversation, including responsiveness, coherence, relevance, topic maintenance etc.

We have already described the loss of phonology and syntax in the previous chapter on primary progressive aphasia. The loss of pragmatic skills of conversation are evident in many cases of the behavioural variety of FTD/Pick's who may not maintain coherent and logical communication, even though other aspects of language appear spared. All these linguistic processes seamlessly intertwine to produce the most important and unique of evolutionary skills, human communication.

Henry Head, a British neurologist, described and coined the term semantic aphasia in the context of head injured soldiers in WW I. Some of these patients with penetrating injuries could neither name nor could they comprehend the meaning of things. Before Head, aphasics who could not name or comprehend yet had fluent speech output were called transcortical (meaning the loss of connections between areas of the brain) sensory aphasics by Wernicke, who systematized aphasiology in the second half of the 19th century, a clinical classification that is still widely

used. A number of cases of these transcortical sensory aphasics were described in the context of progressive degenerative
disease, including one with temporal lobe atrophy by Arnold
Pick in 1904 which was the precursor of this syndrome. The
modern description of the phenomenon was renamed "semantic dementia" in patients with degenerative disorders (Snowden
et al. 1989; Hodges et al. 1992).

The major argument in favour of using the term "dementia" is
that the process extends beyond language to visual recognition
for instance. Transcortical sensory alexia or reading without
meaning, (just like a foreign language text) also accompanies
this syndrome. Furthermore, the individuals afflicted often
complain of forgetting, even though they mean words, not
events. Nevertheless, the decline of semantic processing is
manifested mainly in loss of comprehension and naming of
objects with preserved functioning in other areas of cognition,
in contrast to a global dementing process, such as Alzheimer's
disease. Dementia is an unfortunate label in most instances and
I suspect it will disappear eventually like retardation or imbe-
cility, even from the technical literature.

Considerable amount of shrinkage affecting mainly the left
temporal lobe on neuroimaging is characteristic and indicates a
focal degenerative process in Rita and in other patients (Fig. 3).
The few autopsied cases in progressive semantic aphasia revealed
mostly FTD with MND type pathology, but also Pick's disease
as described in previous chapters. The evidence from "functional" imaging of the normal brain is suggestive for widespread
activation of the cortex for the association of even a single object
with its meaning.[16] Yet, it appears that meaning of objects or

---

16 Functional activation uses isotopes or changes in magnetic resonance signal with increased
blood flow or oxygen utilization in active brain regions during certain cognitive process.

living things can be selectively lost in cases with left temporal lobe atrophy affected by progressive degenerative disease, specifically FTD/Pick complex. Other studies emphasized the involvement of the anterior temporal lobe in herpes encephalitis and head injury in cases where semantic loss occurred for certain categories of objects and nouns with preservation of other language functions. Behavioural abnormality follows the language disorder as a rule when both temporal lobes become affected, as illustrated in the subsequent chapter.

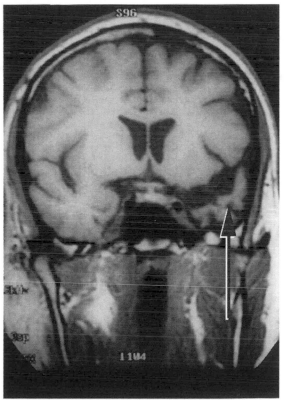

Fig. 3: MRI severe shrinkage of the left temporal lobe (arrow).
Brain is white. Fluid is black. Slice is in the plane of the face. Semantic aphasia.

Colour naming, matching and pointing to colours named were well preserved in Rita, in contrast to aphasics with comprehension deficit due to stroke, as was her ability to calculate and manipulate numbers and to read aloud following the rules of English pronunciation, even though she did not always understand what she was reading. One might argue that this striking preservation of colour, number and letter processing indicates that these concepts are devoid of semantic representation in the same sense as objects, animals, etc. Colours and numbers are attributes of other objects and although their lexical meaning is distinct, they do not by themselves represent independent semantic entities. They can be used as metaphors of course, such as red for revolution or yellow for cowardice, except in semantic dementia. Rita for instance could not choose the right colour for objects or concepts, or discuss the second meaning of certain colours, despite intact visual perception demonstrated by normal performance on the colour blindness (Ishihara) plates and the matching of nonverbal designs.

Although the initial loss of names and comprehension was dependent on the context and the frequency of the words, some items seemed to disappear entirely from her semantic storage and no amount of cueing or changing input modalities could bring them back. Where we store knowledge about objects or persons in our brain is a much researched and largely unsolved issue in neuroscience. The evidence is against conceiving semantic or memory storage for any entity to be located in a single neurone in the cortex. In other words, there is unlikely a single neurone representing a Volkswagen, the "Volkswagen cell" or your grandmother, a "Grandmother cell." The processing of meaning, essential for recognition and associations, depends on the intricate facilitation of the connections of cells established some time ago, something that could no longer be done by Rita's brain.

The so-called lexical (word based) hypothesis of psycholinguistics distinguishes a semantic memory, subserving picture and word meaning processing, which is separate to some extent from a lexicon or a dictionary of words, which can exist without semantic interpretation, let us say for the purpose of pronunciation and writing. Take the example of reading an Italian word like "cacciatore" without knowing the meaning of it. We heard it many times, have seen it in writing, and can order it in a restaurant, taste the sauce, but we still don't know the meaning (I had to look it up in the dictionary: it means "hunter"). Once the relatively finite rules of pronunciation are learned, one can read any word in a foreign language, even though one does not know the meaning of the word. Patients with semantic dementia read English like a foreigner would.

Rita's case clearly supports the separation of assigning meaning (semantic encoding) to objects from other word based (lexical) processes. The preservation of these other lexical processes allowed her to continue to speak fluently, to read, write and repeat words and sentences without meaning! Rita eventually died in a nursing home and her autopsy showed the ubiquinated inclusions typical of the majority of patients with semantic dementia and more than half of the patients with FTD/Pick complex. The next story is also about semantic aphasia or dementia in its more common combination with the behaviour disorder of FTD/Pick's, in a man who became famous for getting away.

Seven

Houdini (Roaming and Restlessness) and the Artist

MALCOLM'S FIRST DIFFICULTY was finding words, such as 'robin', although he could describe it as a red-breasted bird, or 'carnations' when he saw a bunch of flowers or a 'station wagon' when he was trying to talk about one. Later on he did not seem to know the meaning of 'shoe-polish,' 'ice age', or 'asbestos' when these words came up in conversation. Although he was never very good at remembering the names of people, the problem of not being able to recall ordinary words, and furthermore losing their meaning became a puzzling and disturbing symptom.[17] At meetings he did not understand everything that was being said and had to ask his co-workers to elaborate. He remained

---

17 Word finding difficulty can be a normal phenomenon under stress or anxiety, and it can be part of "normal aging" but also an early sign of dementia. It depends on age, associated symptoms and circumstances. By itself it is not very specific, and a minor degree should not alarm people unduly. However, when the meaning of words is gradually lost and the patient does not understand upon hearing, reading, or seeing the object, semantic dementia is said to occur.

competent at tasks requiring visuospatial skills, blueprints, formulae and most nonverbal problem solving tasks, and so his language problems were initially overlooked at work. He was still employed as a professional engineer when I saw him for a neurological assessment. His hobby was carpentry and even though he may have forgotten the name of some of the tools, he had no trouble using them. He built a wall unit as a wedding gift for his son, restored an antique motorcycle and set up and programmed their recently purchased VCR.

Malcolm was a pleasant, handsome man in his early fifties who did not appear to be demented or depressed. His speech output was normal, except for the mild word finding problem and semantic substitutions; for instance, for a bicycle helmet he said, "It's a hat, a safety hat." He had a great deal of trouble recalling the names of persons recently in the news, such as the perpetrator of the Oklahoma bombing or the name of the Premier, even though his memory for events remained intact. In recalling a person, address and flower, he only managed the number of the address but not the street or the names. Subsequently, he was able to recognize some of the items from multiple choices, demonstrating that he in fact registered the names in his short term memory, but he was unable to access them. He did well on serial subtraction, arithmetic and drawing. MRI showed a slight left temporal atrophy and so did the SPECT scan, although these were both read as normal by the radiologist.

On formal neuropsychological testing a year later, he had trouble defining uncommon words, but at times even quite ordinary words were not recognized. He named only about half of the objects presented to him, and he described or gestured the use of some of those he could not name. However, for several items he could not even do that. Not only did he not know what an eggbeater was, he could not show how to use it. Not only its name but its meaning seemed to have disappeared even when it was in front of him and could not be brought back by explanations or relearning. When he read words with irregular spelling that he did not recognize, he would regularize them (island was read "izland" and yacht as "yatcht") as Rita had. Below are examples of his regularization in writing when he was dictated irregular words:

Magician	*magishon*
Biscuit	*biskit*
Salmon	*samon*
Courageous	*corages*
Guile	*gile*
Debt	*det*
Yacht	*yaut*

In contrast to his semantic difficulties he remembered events such as his recent move to London and his daughter's graduation. He continued to drive a car, pay his bills and write cheques, although Alice, his wife, always looked over his shoulder to help. His excellent physical health, relatively preserved memory and visual-spatial orientation allowed him to function. His daughter put his family's pictures with the names beside them in a memory book and they began to compile a dictionary of words he had forgotten. When he went shopping, he read the items off a list, not necessarily knowing their meaning. He also reported impaired recognition of voices on the telephone (called "auditory agnosia"). In fact, he seemed to have the same extraordinary disorder as Rita with one important exception.

Two years after his initial visit, he developed a set of behavioural symptoms, so distressing to his wife that it was she who was admitted to a psychiatric unit with a depressive breakdown. This was precipitated by Malcolm's altering their basement in order to put up his huge jigsaw puzzle pictures, despite her efforts to dissuade him. Malcolm developed other compulsive routines and food fads such as insisting on eating Chinese food every time they passed a food court in a mall or having doughnuts instead of a proper lunch. He was childish about trying to get the largest doughnut and pouted if he thought he got a smaller one. He put a great deal of plum sauce on rice, excessive maple syrup on pancakes, and went back for several helpings of Chinese food. On several occasions, he drove some 200 kilometres to a doughnut shop in their old neighbourhood and 85 kilometres to a fish and chip restaurant, 85 kilometres in the other direction.

Contrary to his previous taste in entertainment, he was into watching old John Wayne or Arnold Schwarzenegger movies. "The Price is Right" or "Wheel of Fortune" fascinated him and he tried to get his wife to watch them too. However, he was unable to pay attention to more complex stories and would get up after a few minutes. His reasoning seemed to be affected and it was hard to explain anything to him. Although his grammar was intact and he remained surprisingly fluent, when he did not understand and just perseverated, Alice showed frustration, and he could perceive this. In turn, she would feel intensely guilty afterwards. She joined our Pick's disease support group, which helped her to cope.[18]

On his third and last visit his speech was still relatively fluent, but he had a great deal of trouble comprehending single words, even common ones such as pencil, cup, and comb. He could not point to these even when he had only six to choose from. On the other hand, he had no problems pointing to letters, numbers, or colours (see the discussion on Rita for the reason for the preservation of the mental processing in these categories). His naming difficulty was equally severe. He could only name a knife, spoon and fork out of 20 items and his naming did not improve on tactile cues. Although he could read sentences he did not always know their meaning.[19] He could repeat well, even material he could not comprehend.

Malcolm's compulsive roaming and driving became his undoing. His wife and the rest of the family tried all avenues of persuasion and distraction, only to meet with stubborn resistance and anger, completely out of character. Everyone agreed that formal suspension of his licence would not deter him and eventually, they took his keys away. He resorted to hot-wiring his ignition, and on another occasion, he was ready to drive away in someone else's car, which had the key left in the ignition while the driver paid gas. The police were called and Alice hurried to the scene to deal with the situation. The next time, he managed to drive away in a stranger's car, a "swat team" was called. Fortunately they noticed his

---

18 Support groups for Pick's disease sufferers and their families have been formed in the United Kingdom, United States, Canada, France, and Germany. Recently, an international association for caregivers of FTD has been established, called "The Association for Frontotemporal Dementias," Website: www.ftd-picks.org

19 His reading, characterized by errors of regularizations and semantic substitutions, is also described as surface dyslexia by linguists since the meaning, or the surface structure of language is lost in contrast to the preserved grammar and morphology which are surface structures.

medic-alert bracelet and Malcolm ended up in the closed ward of the psychiatric hospital. He learned the door code quickly through his superior visual-spatial skills by watching the staff punch in the numbers, and eventually handle covers had to be used to control this. He then used windows to exit. He would take food away from other people and even when he was tied to a chair he would get up with the chair on his back and move around. The nurses started to refer to him affectionately as Houdini.

A particularly frequent and disrupting form of disinhibited compulsive behaviour is the frequent roaming and restlessness that may take the form of walking miles and miles to go to a mall or just around the neighbourhood, or of driving long distances to a favourite location. Caregivers may become concerned about the safety of the roamer, but restriction of this activity is often met with resistance and anger. FTD patients resemble to some extent children with attention deficit and hyperactivity disorder who carry the symptoms with them into adulthood, but the behaviour change in FTD develops in middle age. Activity and attention levels are much studied phenomena in neuroscience and are related to certain structures such as the brainstem and the thalamus which alerts and activates us. The limbic circuit, particularly the cingulate gyrus in the inner surface of the frontal lobes, modulates directed attention and activity. The frontal cortex contributes both the maintenance and inhibition of activity levels and these modulating influences seem to be deficient in FTD patients. Examples of restlessness and roaming from caregivers:

...Roams the neighborhood and invites herself in...goes to the mall with a seniors' group and roams until night when everything is closed...drives to Toronto to see her sister daily... walks for miles to visit his wife at work twice a day...can't sit still...drives to Detroit and California without explaining why...became obsessed with walking ... drives to the legion daily...drives his car around without any purpose...found walking on the highway by police... walks and drives excessively...paces up and down the halls...drives around without a licence...wanders a lot...unable to stay still...out of the house every day...wanders outside...wanders off during the night...attempts to leave the house...very restless, paces a lot...gets up and down from the dinner table...goes out in the middle of the night...has to walk every day...gets up in the middle of the interview to walk around...spends much of her day walking...walks restlessly around stores without buying anything...he does not stay put very long...wants to go out in the car all the time...gets up and walks around during meals...goes and sits in the car until his wife takes him somewhere...power walks to exhaustion...wants to go places all the time...

Malcolm's illness, like Rita's, also began with "semantic aphasia" like Rita's, but his behavioural disturbance appeared earlier and more prominently. Although many aspects of semantic dementia have been studied in detail, especially by John Hodges and his associates in Cambridge, because of the selectivity of the deficit and the intriguing contrast to a more diffuse dementia and other language deficits, its association with the behavioural disorder has not been emphasized. A degree of semantic dementia is relatively common with the behavioural presentation of FTD/Pick's. Isolated instances of persisting semantic dementia without the behavioural disorder, such as in Rita in the chapter "What is Steak?" are actually unusual. The semantic loss often goes beyond the language modality, as these patients may not recognize objects visually. The subsequent development of bizarre behaviour is another reason the term "dementia" is used, although semantic aphasia may be preferable as being more specific and less negative.

Malcolm's case actually contradicts the classic dogma of the famous French neurologist Pierre Marie that intelligence is impaired in aphasia. Marie's well known example was a French chef who could not make an omelette after his aphasic stroke. Failing to make an omelette may not be as much a loss of general intelligence, but could be attributed to apraxia or a failure of planned motor activity that often accompanies aphasia. Although language interacts with and supports many aspects of cognition, the relative independence of language from other instrumental modalities of cognition has been repeatedly demonstrated in experiments, including our previous studies with stroke aphasics. It was, in fact, Malcolm's remarkably preserved visuospatial intelligence and a strong desire to roam that made his behaviour a constant challenge to his caregivers.

Compulsive playing of games or creation of jigsaw puzzles is common and occupies considerable time of the patients in early stages. Some patients become doodlers and the occasional individual may take up painting, some with artistic merit, indicating that disinhibition may even release artistic expression and preoccupation with creative tools and crafts may produce, albeit temporarily, positive results. Dr. Bruce Miller, from San Francisco, has shown this paradox with several interesting patients and their colourful paintings (Miller et al. 1998). I had two patients like this myself, one who had been an accomplished artist, and who continued drawing late into her illness (Fig. 4). The other one who

took up water colours after her illness began. Others complete
huge jigsaw pictures, like Malcolm or Keith, or play word games
day in and day out. Eventually inattention, apathy or restlessness,
and deterioration of manual and language skills terminate the
creative activity, which may have been a welcome respite from
physical compulsions and perseverative routines.

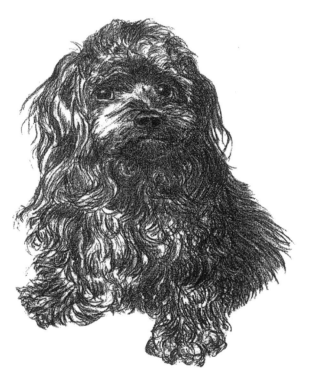

Fig. 4: Drawing by a patient with semantic dementia and well preserved
artistic ability.

Jill, the 61 year old artist who drew Fig. 4, also had
semantic dementia at the time she created the picture. She
came to see me because she could not remember names.

Her husband told us she did not know the meaning of words such as "horseradish" and "refrigerator". She could not follow conversation because she could not understand complex topics. She also developed personality changes, such as inflexibility and stubbornness often "getting a bee in her bonnet". She became extra sensitive to pets, adoring them in a childish, gushy manner. She also appeared more forward with people, expressed opinions about things she did not know much about and furthermore was adamant and argumentative about it. She had left temporal atrophy like Rita and eventually she had to be admitted to a nursing home because of her unmanageable obsessions and marital breakdown.

Like Malcolm (Houdini) she learned the spatial pattern of the 5 sequence security pad in use instead of keys in the nursing home, by observing the nurses' hand movements. She stopped drawing, but she can still put together huge 1000 piece jigsaw puzzles in two days. Her husband thinks that her colour discrimination has become more sensitive and she picks up matching colours faster than anybody else. Her language became impoverished, but she would still talk fluently about religion: "God has promised paradise on earth, and Jesus is going to heal me (pointing to her forehead) in the Kingdom of Heaven." Yet, a few minutes later she may ask: "What is Kingdom?" when she hears the words "Kingdom Hall" from someone else.

Eight

The Alien Hand
(Extrapyramidal Symptoms)

THE THIRD COMPONENT of FTD/Pick's was not recognized for a while as part of the same illness and there is still a debate going on about just where it belongs. Now it is increasingly being considered an entity that straddles both the domain of movement and cognitive disorders. Described first by a group of Harvard physicians as a separate variety of Parkinson's disease, it was considered a "Parkinson Plus" syndrome and classified among the disorders of the extrapyramidal motor system. The complex neural circuit modulating movements is called extrapyramidal, because it is in addition (extra) to the main motor (pyramidal) pathway of direct connection between the cortex and the spinal cord. The most commonly recognized disorder of the extrapyramidal system is Parkinson's disease. The plus designation, which is still used by many physicians to express a difference, came from the recognition of additional features, such as the severe apraxia, the strange, "alien hand" and the lack of typical Parkinsonian tremor. As neurologists began to recognize the illness, they renamed it corticobasal degeneration (CBD), because the disease affected the cortex as well as the base of the brain. An increasing number of cases, including the original ones, were described with cognitive and behavioural disorders, particularly aphasia. Interestingly, the original authors which included one of the best neuropathologists at Harvard, E.P. Richardson, remarked that the histology most resembled Pick's disease, particularly the abundance of ballooned neurons or "Pick cells" (Rebeiz et al. 1964). However, the disease remained mainly in the domain of the movement disorder specialists and up to this day the issue of classification has continued to be controversial. The last three conferences on FTD however accepted CBD as part of the Pick complex. The following story is an example of this strange combination of cognitive, behavioural and movement disorder featuring the "alien hand."

Chris, a 63-year-old, right-handed engineer, developed stiffness in his right arm shortly after his second marriage. His writing deteriorated and he was unable to control his lawnmower. Six months later he was holding his right arm at his side, like a stroke victim and he started to lose balance. It was as if gravity seemed to propel him forward. About the same time, his speech diminished, he had word finding difficulty, and he lost interest in friends and daily activities. He became perseverative with words and ideas and had difficulty organizing complex activities. His thought process seemed to have slowed down and he had trouble with sequential actions. Parkinson's disease was diagnosed but Levodopa, which often works wonders in that disease, and some other Parkinson medications were ineffective.

A year after onset it was noted that his right hand was interfering with his left, as if it belonged to someone else: "an alien hand." His right hand was clumsy and useless. On examination he was very apractic, literally lacking practice, meaning that he could not perform skilled movements or gestures. Not only could not carry them out on command, even though he had no trouble comprehending and responding verbally, but he could not imitate them either. A CT scan showed left parietal atrophy as in Fig. 2. The parietal lobe is considered to be responsible for sensori-motor integration and damage to it often results in apraxia among other symptoms.

As he progressed, he was noted to be apathetic, slow, and aphasic. His right hand showed unusual posturing but he seemed to ignore it. The diagnosis of corticobasal degeneration syndrome (CBDS) was made about two and a half years after onset. His behaviour and personality started to change also. Although he remained polite in public, he became preoccupied with sex, watching erotic videos, masturbating, and demanding sex daily. His speech became aphasic, he searched for words, used phrases unrelated to the discussion and he could not put a sentence together. He became angry and frustrated when he was not understood.

About three years after onset he became incontinent of urine. His right leg became stiff and the fingers of his right hand curled. Six months later he was admitted to a chronic care hospital and had to be fed since he could not use his right arm. Later, he became mute and his swallowing was impaired, but he could still yell when upset. He responded to teasing with a giggle, he still watched television, tapped his foot to music, and licked his lips when he watched "Electric Circus." He cried on hearing familiar songs and when his minister visited. He died nine years after onset, following a urinary tract infection and sepsis at the age of 74. Just before his death, he had bilateral rigidity, severe immobility, vertical gaze palsy, and total mutism on neurological examination.

On autopsy the brain showed marked atrophy of the frontal and parietal lobes, and moderate atrophy of the temporal lobe, slightly more on the left side. Microscopic examination showed ring shaped neuronal inclusions typical of Corticobasal Degeneration (CBD). Abnormal "Tau protein" was abundant in the glia (see the biology chapter for the significance of Tau)[20] and ballooned neurons (Pick cells) were scattered in the cortex. Chris' case is an example of a CBD syndrome (CBDS) diagnosed in life, soon followed by the onset of behavioural symptoms of FTD and later progressive aphasia, and finally confirmed CBD pathology.

Clinical descriptions of CBDS, usually from movement disorder clinics, have emphasized motor manifestations, such as one sided rigidity, apraxia and the alien hand syndrome. The alien hand phenomenon refers to a hand moving or feeling strange as if it did not belong to the person. One of the earliest description came from Kurt Goldstein, a German neurologist, who presented a woman, with a stroke which had destroyed some of the pathways between the two halves of the brain,

---

20 A proliferation of the glial cells, forming a scar, is a common reaction to many types of injury in the brain, but a particularly characteristic feature of Pick's disease/FTD. Glial cells were considered to provide mainly structural and metabolic support in the brain, but their function in neural transmission is increasingly recognized.

called the corpus callosum. She tried to choke herself with her left hand while the right hand tried to restrain the "alien left", much like Peter Sellers in "Dr Strangelove" trying to pull down his artificial arm from a habitual, uncontrollable Nazi salute. Further descriptions of one hand interfering with another came after surgically separating the hemispheres of the brain to stop the spread of epilepsy (sectioning the corpus callosum). The expression "alien hand" was subsequently adopted to describe some of the motor deficit in CBDS. True intermanual conflict, or one hand actually interfering with the other is unusual, but unilateral motor neglect, rigidity and a levitating (the hand floats up in the air), clumsy, useless hand are common.

A different variety of alien hand is frequently encountered in cases of severe neglect, usually associated with a large right hemispheric stroke. Such patients do not feel that the paralysed left hand or leg belongs to them, and they confabulate about it, claiming that the nurses put it there, or somebody else left it. The alien limb is perceived as foreign, ugly, rotten, or dead and may be called various nicknames by the patient. Macdonald Critchley, the most erudite of descriptive British neurologists, collected some of these: "Monkey", "Silly Billy", "Floppy Joe", "Gammy", "the Curse", "Lazy Bones" etc. An extreme variety of this phenomenon is dramatized by Oliver Sacks in his collection of essays about neurological patients, "The Man Who Mistook His Wife for a Hat." One of his stroke patients threw his "alien hand" out of the bed and fell out of the bed after it. This extent of delusional depersonalization is not seen in the "motor alien hand" of CBDS, although the patients often complain that the hand behaves as if it did not belong to them, but had a mind of its own. This raises the interesting philosophical issue of what is "free will", and what is an uncontrollable reflex action, an argument elegantly discussed by Miller Fisher in the context of the "Alien Hand". It is argued that all of our actions represent a reaction, a reflex to a stimulus. However, many of our conscious actions are accompanied by a sense of our willing them.

Alien hand is an exception that is all the more striking because the movements are similar to other willed movements, rather than reflexes. An item about alien hand is part of our Frontal Behavioral Inventory (FBI) because it may not be obvious on examination, but caregivers who have had a greater opportunity to observe it, may be able to recall the onset and extent of it.

Nine

The Hero of Bolero
(Supranuclear Palsy)

M Y "HERO OF BOLERO" was Dudley Moore, the
British comic actor, playing a composer who falls
in love with the "perfect woman" in the movie "10." The
musical theme of that memorable movie was Ravel's catchy
composition of perfection, "Bolero". Dudley Moore died
relatively young of progressive supranuclear palsy (PSP),
which is the subject of our next story. Coincidentally,
Ravel also died with progressive aphasia, which is a related condition. A few people are beginning to realize that
PSP has a great deal in common with CBD and the FTD/
Pick complex, and that it should be considered part of it.
Perhaps the majority of physicians and even specialists are
still not aware and others are not willing to recognize the
extent of the association, and continue to believe strongly
that they are different diseases, for various reasons. Not
that this discussion is unique to PSP and FTD. The same

debate appears for instance in considering the relation of Dementia with Parkinson's disease and the "Lewy body variant" of Alzheimer's disease. The "splitters" and the "lumpers" continue to argue how diseases should be classified, named and defined in many other areas of medicine and biology, but especially in new and technologically advancing territory.

Carlo is 68 when he is referred because of suspected frontotemporal dementia, a diagnosis made by a geriatrician in another town. By the time he comes to see me, he has something else. It is not that the geriatrician made the wrong diagnosis. On the contrary, he was one hundred percent right. Carlo's history, as you will surely recognize as you read on, is typical of FTD/Pick's, but his difficulty walking is not. Not, if they are considered different diseases. He pushes a walker in front of him. Without it, he shuffles with short steps and has a hard time initiating movements. When he gets going, he propels himself forward faster and faster with shortening steps ("festination" as neurologists call it). At other times he falls backward and has to step back in order to stay upright. He turns his body rigidly in a block, like a robot and has difficulty getting up on the examining table or getting out of a chair.

He can not look up and down and can not follow a finger with his eyes sideways; in technical terms he has "vertical gaze palsy and impaired horizontal pursuit." When he wants to look at his watch, he has to raise his arm up in front of his eyes. This is the "watch salute," I tell my residents, so they will remember the signature symptom, which is the vertical gaze palsy giving the disease

its name. He bursts out crying or laughs with no provocation (also known as "pseudobulbar palsy").[21] He may
start with a chuckle which blends into a sobbing cry. His
smile appears forced and spastic, resembling the fixed,
sardonic grin of tetanus cramps ("rhisus sardonicus"), and
his speech is slow and slurred, with a strange singsong
inflection. A rapid jerky tremor is evident in the right
hand, especially when he is moving, writing or drawing,
not the typical tremor of Parkinson's disease. His writing
is small, micrographic. When he is asked to draw a clock,
the outlining circle is minuscule, the numbers are crowded
together and difficult to recognize. He fails to place the
hands appropriately.

Most experienced neurologists would diagnose Progressive Supranuclear Palsy at this point, but his illness started
approximately four years before, with errors in judgment
while driving and careless handling of money. He made
wide turns, drove with his car trunk open, drove on to lawns
and curbs and he would suddenly stop unnecessarily, much
before coming to a stop sign. Eventually he rear-ended
somebody and when got into another accident a year later,
drifting into another lane, he lost his licence. In the last two
years socially inappropriate behaviour, rudeness and short
attention span appeared. He would get up during the middle of a conversation and leave. He called his daughter and
granddaughter "bitches" without reason. He would not wait
for mealtime, but would often reach for a can of beans and
eat out of the can. He developed an obsession for salami ,
eating a half-pound at once, directly from the package.

---

21 "Bulbar" means, that the innervation of muscles involved in swallowing, speaking, laughing
and crying originate in the bulb shaped part of the brainstem. Pseudobulbar means that other
structures outside the "bulb" are affected causing impaired function in the same muscles

He compulsively watched TV from 6:30 p.m. until midnight, while neglecting his chores. He stopped doing yard work and his personal hygiene was also slipping, wearing the same clothes for a week at a time and only showering at the YMCA twice a week, after his exercise. When asked, he shaved with an electric shaver, while sitting watching TV, otherwise he walked around with stubble on his face. He would not put on socks, arguing it was unnecessary while he was wearing his shoes. His wife discovered he was hiding cash in the basement. Others in the family noticed he was often fidgety, manipulating objects for no reason. He also became emotionally distant, disinterested and only talked about what he watched on television. Later, he stopped participating in conversation, and had difficulty getting words out. His customers at his shop, which had become quite messy, noticed his lack of patience and easy frustration.

The geriatrician observed that he was impulsive and interrupted conversations with unrelated thoughts and concerns. He had trouble with some of the sequential motor tests and similarities, which are considered "executive function". A CAT scan showed some mild frontoparietal atrophy and the diagnosis of early frontotemporal dementia was made. The movement disorder became evident several years after the behavioural symptoms. He was still working, leaning against the counter and moving around with some difficulty, but when he began having trouble turning around and started falling, he had to stop. A rapid tremor developed in the right hand, especially when he was agitated. He continued being impulsive, impatient and restless. At a restaurant he would finish his meal, leave and wait beside the car until his family was ready to take him home. He was emotional and tearful,

at times with no provocation. His speech became perseverative and slurred, less intelligible. He often repeated words
and only spoke in short sentences.

My former professor of neurology in Toronto, J.C.
Richardson, and a then fellow resident and good friend John
Steele described a form of "Parkinson-plus" syndrome associated with gaze palsy, falling, slurred speech, "pseudobulbar" crying/laughing, and choking and called it "progressive
supranuclear palsy" (PSP) (Steele et al 1964). The neuropathologist was Jerzy Olszewski, one of the best in his field.
John Steele, the only surviving member of the team, is now
living on the Pacific island of Guam, treating and studying
the strange combination of ALS-Parkinsonism-Dementia
of the native Chamorros; his life there as the "Gaugin of
Neurology" is eloquently described by Oliver Sacks in his
book: "The Island of the Colour Blind".

The movement disorder which the islanders call "Lytico-
Bodig" resembles PSP, according to John Steele. Some
of the patients look like the immobile postencephalitic
Parkinsonian catatonics, who were treated by Oliver Sacks,
and whose story was dramatized in the book and the film
"Awakenings". The pathology in the islanders is essentially
a tauopathy having features of Alzheimer's, PSP and post
encephalitic parkinsonism. More about this geographic
cluster of neurodegeneration resembling PSP in combination with ALS (Amyotrophic Lateral Sclerosis) can be found
in Chapter 14.

Steele, Richardson and Olszewski pointed out the unique
features of PSP, separating it from Parkinson's disease.
Dudley Moore was one of the famous people dying with

PSP, providing it a "face" to lift it from obscurity, and there are large, well-organized advocacy groups championing it as a unique "orphan "disease. The behavioural disorder and progressive aphasia is infrequently mentioned, although relatively commonly associated. Cognitive symptoms featured prominently in the original description by Steele et al. and in other papers ever since. Some investigators consider it the prototype of "subcortical dementia", yet many regard it as a movement disorder only. True enough, not all cases of PSP develop the behavioural symptoms so typical of FTD as did Carlo, and those who have the movement disorder first, may be too incapacitated and immobile to manifest it or may die from one of their choking spells. On the other hand, many FTD patients have "PSP like symptoms" later in their illness (See Chapters 4, 7, 17, and 19). Many become progressively dysarthric (slurred speech), aphasic, and mute, developing the language component of Pick complex.

The other day I got a call from D. B., a friend of mine and an excellent neuro-ophthalmologist in Montreal (these specialists often see PSP because of the striking up and down gaze disturbance), saying: "I have seen a woman with PSP, who says you have treated other members of her family with frontotemporal dementia, but she seems to have a different disease". She turned out to be a cousin of Rachel, Becky, and Gordon from Chapters 11-13. Interestingly, the typical neuropathology in this family is not PSP, but the ubiquitin staining neuronal inclusions of motor neurone disease (ALS) In other families with FTD there are individuals in whom the first symptoms suggest PSP. Does this mean that there are two different neurodegenerative disorders appearing in the same family? Not necessarily, it is more likely that they are different presentations of the same illness. It is also likely that the seemingly different ALS and PSP pathology are related more than was previously believed, possibly providing a clue to the cause of these illnesses. Recently, the discovery of mutations in the progranulin gene in families with tau negative pathology on chromosome 17, where tau is located, also suggests a relationship (see discussion on the biology in the "Lost and Found" chapter.

There is considerable research into the basic biology of PSP, which shows an identical abnormality of the tau protein to what was found in corticobasal degeneration (CBD). Without going into unnecessary detail, an excess of a certain type of protein called 4 repeat (4R) tau is common to both. Genetic and histochemical studies also indicate a considerable overlap. Time and again, we find that they have common clinical features and we designate this variety of Pick complex as CBD/PSP. A patient, for instance, was referred to me as a case of CBD by another neurologist, but the movement disorder specialist at our centre thought the symptoms were more typical of PSP. We argued about the diagnosis back and forth, recognizing the close relationship of the two all the while. The pathology turned out to be CBD, but even the pathologists have arguments about distinguishing the two. The differences are a matter of emphasis.

There is increasing evidence that the typical PSP pathology can occur with progressive aphasia, or the behavioural disorder and that PSP symptoms occur with other varieties of pathology within the Pick complex. This creates confusion among caregivers and even among doctors, not up to date on the arguments about the diagnostic distinctions. A caregiver is justified to ask: "How come the pathology report says CBD when we were told he had PSP?" The answer is that the cases are similar in life and arguably difficult to distinguish even on postmortem examination. They may be best looked at as variant manifestations of the same disease.

Ten

The Sexy Senior (Hypersexuality)

WHEN GWEN'S GRAVELLY voice and cackle fills the waiting room, I scramble to get her in my office, because she puts on quite a show and often shocks other unsuspecting patients waiting there. She sings little ditties, shakes her torso provocatively and bumps her hips against me when I go out to greet her. Her daughters are apologetic, embarrassed and angry at the same time. Their desperation is often voiced, "We just don't know what to do with her," as they provide a story of bizarre behaviour characterized by disinhibition and poor judgment, which is becoming steadily worse. She is a 72-year-old woman living on her own, requiring an increasing amount of supervision, because of the serious social and personal consequences of her behaviour.

Her oldest daughter remembered: "The first time we were concerned was about five years ago when she joined a dance club and bought a cruise with the club for $14,000. This was about three times as much as she should have paid, because it included the cost of an "escort". We called the Better Business Bureau and prevented the deal from going through. We also notified the police, who spoke with mom explaining why it was not a good idea to go. She told us the police said, "Oh, go ahead." She later went on another cruise with her grandson and a friend and boasted, "Everybody thought I was having sex with him." More recently, she had invited a 38-year-old man, who was installing some windows for her, to go to Mexico with her and we had to intervene and get her money back, because she had already bought the tickets for both of them. She became obsessed with sexual matters and talked about it constantly. Out of the blue she asked her grandson, "How does a lesbian make love?" This behaviour had become so embarrassing that her grandchildren avoided her company.

Her poor judgment about money and sex created continous upheaval. She let another strange young man into her home, who persuaded her to buy $6,000 worth of cold storage equipment, again prevented with some difficulty by her daughters. They estimated she had gone through about $100,000 of her nest egg. As a result of these confrontations she believed, not entirely unreasonably from her point of view, that her daughters were after her money and wanted to put her in a nursing home.

An equally, if not more alarming, problem was her driving, which became erratic: she was changing lanes without looking behind, once driving on the shoulder thinking it was a lane especially for her. She clipped someone's side mirror but she talked herself out of the situation.

Another time, when she went through a red light, hitting two other cars, she insisted she did not, but her daughters read the accident report. For some reason she was never charged. They noticed her having trouble putting her car in gear and she had difficulty regulating the thermostat at home.

Her manners deteriorated shockingly. On one occasion her grandson answered the phone and asked if she wanted to leave a message, she replied: "Oh, go to hell." She would be rude to strangers and would ask a person in front of her in a line, "What are you buying this for?" She stared at people, making faces and sticking her tongue out at them, and made racist comments about somebody wearing a turban. She was irritable, easily angered, told her daughters off and was unwilling to go along with their suggestions. She neglected her hygiene, did not wash her hands, changed her clothes infrequently and failed to clean her house. At times the toilet seat was soiled.

In my office, she displays a great deal of bizarre behaviour. She is overly familiar and keeps repeating, "I'm sure you think I am nuts." She is rude to her daughters, calling them "nuts," and saying "baloney" to everything they say. I soon have to separate them. During examination, she wiggles herself in a suggestive manner and appears quite distractible. In contrast to her bizarre behaviour, she is fully oriented, has no language difficulty and although she loses points on impulsive drawing and inattentiveness, her Mini Mental State Exam score is still a borderline high of 26/30. Despite this, I have no choice but to report her driving errors to the Province of Ontario, which obliges doctors to do so, when safety becomes a concern.

After she lost her driver's licence she walked a lot, sometimes on the railroad track, other times on the shoulder of the highway. She seemed unwilling to use a taxi. Impulsively, she joined a golf club, but did not play much, her daughters heard, because she was swearing and people avoided her. She frequented the legion hall, getting up to dance and flirt. Her daughters were particularly upset on finding that she had taken a younger man in his 50's, an alcoholic whom she had met at the legion, home with her and had him sleep in her bed. She seemed unable to perceive the possible consequences of certain situations. There were also concerns about her health and safety, because she reused old supermarket bags that chicken had been wrapped in. Food accumulated in her fridge and went bad. She had stereotypic food habits, always buying a couple of potatoes, a couple of bananas, one apple, and "fig Newtons". Her daughters initiated Meals-On-Wheels and a cleaning lady and they would look in on her whenever she let them.

When I saw her for the third year in a row she had lost some weight. Her language was still quite fluent, although inappropriately facetious and coarse. She had a teasing, smart-alecky patter, but she was angry with me because she remembered I had something to do with the loss of her licence. She now displayed mild semantic aphasia or difficulty with the meaning of words (See the chapter on, "What is Steak?"). This consisted of the inability to understand or define infrequently used nouns such as zebra or jar, or to name them when shown a picture. She was still oriented and aware of recent events, although somewhat circumstantial and concrete. Sometimes she just ignored questions and kept talking about something else.

Nine years into her illness, she was admitted to a psychiatric institution because of decreasing comprehension and
inability to organize her daily activities. She could not prepare a meal and sometimes put the dishes away unwashed
or incompletely cleaned. When transferred to a nursing
home, she adjusted to the new environment and began
playing euchre and bingo. She was reading books, but her
daughters doubted she understood them. A mild tranquil-
izer helped her restlessness and agitation.

This patient and many others with FTD display a disturb-
ingly disinhibited hypersexuality. There is a resemblance to
the behaviour of the bilateral temporal lobectomies in the
Kluver-Bucy experiments. In middle-aged or older individuals hypersexuality is often verbal rather than an actual increase
in libido, but occasionally there is increased initiation of overt
sexual activity from both sexes. Mostly, it is associated with
other forms of disinhibition and poor judgment. Preoccupation
with genitalia, breasts, and bras are particularly common (see
the chapter "The Bra Obsession"). Some just talk about it
incessantly or make risqué jokes or comments. Others touch
strangers, peer into their cleavage or lift their dresses. Sexually
charged jokes overlap with another variety of disinhibition,
related to frontal lesions and described as inappropriate jocularity, or "witzelsucht" (translated as a flood of jokes: see the
chapters on "Moria" and "Sister Act"). Some may walk around
the house in various stages of undress, in front of their families.
Actual sexual activity, if still performed, is often diminished,
quick and without feeling, foreplay, or consideration. Spouses
feel horrified, disgusted, rejected and angry at having to cope
with this unwelcome change. This behaviour in public is so

bizarre and out of context that it is rarely perceived as dangerous molestation, and tends to elicit embarrassment or pity with the exception being if directed towards children. Hypersexuality is at times seen with right frontal or anterior temporal tumors or strokes and in a few patients who are receiving Levodopa or Dopamine agonists for Parkinson's disease.

There were many patients in my practice with FTD who display similar hypersexuality:

...Makes sexual comments and jokes, asks his grandchildren about their sex lives..."I can't lie flat because my boobs stick up"... makes inappropriate sexual innuendos towards male strangers, flirts in doctor's office...talks about sex a lot...sexually inappropriate with a male resident in her nursing home...has called 1-900 numbers (telephone sex), makes sexual remarks...talks about her sex life to an employee of her husband...asked her husband for sex nightly, claiming that it helped her to sleep... appears half-naked in front of family, obsessed with breasts and bras, makes sexual comments to grandchildren, asks her son-in-law if her boobs looked alright?... obsessed with sexual matters and talks about sex constantly... interested in other people's sex lives...makes jokes with a sexual connotation, has increased sexual desires...touches himself a lot, would like to "do it" daily...flirtatious in an inappropriate way...obsessed with pictures of teenage boys... crawls into other people's beds, acting out sexually...tries to get "friendly" with people...started asking family members about their sex lives; tried to make out with his wife while shopping...tells people she is "not getting anything," lifted up her shirt to show people her bra...makes explicit sexual suggestions to strange females in public...sexually aggressive...looks at pornographic material constantly...said to a stranger in a store: "my husband likes me naked..."

Gwen's story also illustrates the financial, ethical, and emotional conflicts caregivers may encounter. Her daughters found themselves in an impossible situation. They felt she needed protection from the consequences of her poor judgment in finances, driving, and personal relationships, but she did not want any of it. Many such patients are paranoid about their relatives' or caregivers' efforts to prevent impulsive or ill considered spending. Sometimes they believe that the relatives just want to inherit more money and sometimes this assignment of motivation may seem reasonable. Physicians and associated health workers are often placed in the middle of a conflict because of these financial issues. Since they are patient advocates, independence or financial autonomy is not taken away from patients lightly..[22] Poor judgment may not be clear and patients often manage to rationalize. Usually not until other manifestations of social inappropriateness are evident, is incompetence acknowledged or officially declared. Furthermore, these patients often have relatively intact cognition and screening tests for dementia, such as the MMSE, may be within normal limits. Certification of incompetence requires increasingly stringent criteria in most jurisdictions and specially trained examiners in some, while a letter from a physician may have sufficed in the past.

Gwen had other typical features of FTD/Pick's disease such as stereotypic food habits (but not gluttony), compulsive roaming and neglect of her household and personal hygiene. Later on in her illness she had features of semantic language disorder (see chapters on "What is Steak?" and "Houdini").

---

22 It is generally useful and highly recommended to obtain a Power of Attorney for all issues including finances early, before illness develops, because competency examinations and legal procedures to solve these problems can be costly and difficult.

It was the deterioration of her living conditions to a state of squalor that eventually led to her hospitalization. Her male counterpart is described in the next chapter.

Eleven

Man in the Barrel (Senile Squalor)

G REGORY WAS THE MALE counterpart of Gwen, mirroring her age and behaviours even though they had never met. He was a dashing young hero of WWII, rising to the rank of major in one of the partisan armies of Eastern Europe. In Canada he worked as a civil and mechanical engineer and had retired 11 years before being seen, divorcing his first wife at that time. Always a dapper man, fond of good clothes, gourmet food and dancing, he acquired a girlfriend and moved in with her after a couple of years. He was a big spender and liked to cook fancy meals for her[23]. Trouble began when he started to neglect himself; sometimes he would not wash, make his own bed or clean his room. He had to be reminded to change his

---

23 He could have served as a model for the European hero of "The Book of Eve" by Beresford-Howe. The middle-aged, "WASP" heroine of this book leaves her secure slavery to a crippled, but tyrannical husband and after being on her own she moves in with an eccentric and romantic Hungarian.

clothes and to bathe. He left everything out, the pots and pans on the burners, and the dishes in the sink. When the sink got full, he put his dirty dishes into the bathtub and promised to hire somebody to clean up. Once he caused a small fire during one of his grand culinary productions and his lady friend made him move into a separate apartment in the same building. She became aware of his inappropriate and impulsive spending and an outstanding credit card balance of $34,000. He bought 100 sheets of plywood on speculation, but did not arrange storage. For three weeks, he spent $100 a day on lottery tickets. He spent $600 on telephone sex. He began calling her about trivial matters seven or eight times a day. He bought a large dog and left him on the balcony with food but no water. The barking created a commotion and the Humane Society came to take the dog away.

His lady friend recalled that he had liked to "talk dirty" with a lot of sexual innuendos for years before things got out of hand, but lately he became quite indiscriminate about what he said or to whom. His sex drive increased and he talked about it and about his girlfriend's body to friends and strangers. Previously well dressed and fastidious, who used to wear his tuxedo on every possible occasion, he now appeared in the local corner store in his slippers and a housecoat loosely secured with nothing under it. On other occasions, he went down to his girlfriend's apartment wearing only a pair of satin boxer shorts and often removed all of his clothes at her place. In the summer, he slept nude on the balcony.

For many years he had been in the habit of taking the sugar packets from restaurants, rationalizing that he had paid for them. Once, when out with his lady friend, he tried to take the mustard container. Finally, he was caught removing products from her workplace, arrested and taken to court, but he was not convicted. His smoking became unsafe; he burned several holes in her furniture. When he moved to his own apartment she sent all the furniture, with cigarette burns, with him. He started drinking compulsively after he heard on television that a couple of drinks a day were good for your health. He helped himself to a concoction of raisins soaked in gin 9-10 times per day and said that this improved his arthritis.

Although he maintained he has never had an accident driving, she gave examples where he had bumped into other cars and he had actually backed into hers on one occasion. He would minimize the problem, saying they were minor things due to mechanical failure of his brakes. His grandchildren were terrified to go with him in the car since he was smoking at the same time he was driving. After several scrapes his licence was suspended, but he continued to drive his vintage Cadillac and Mustang and bought nine bicycles.

At a geriatric assessment his cognition was normal on screening tests and he was considered rational and competent financially. His behaviour was attributed to vascular disease of the brain, because of white spots on the MRI.[24] Three months later the police picked him up for urinating in public and took him to the emergency department for a psychiatric evaluation. He also soiled himself at a restaurant and this was attributed to previously diagnosed bowel

24 These white spots, hyperintensities, or UBOs (unidentified bright objects) often appear in normal aging and their significance continues to be debated. They are often over-interpreted as the cause of disease.

problems (diverticulosis), or alternatively and more likely to his consumption of large quantities of olive and sunflower oil with salad or bread.

When the geriatric psychiatry team assessed him at home, his apartment was in total disarray, with clothing, boxes, plastic bags, and other material strewn all over. There were dishes piled high in the sink and the bathtub and the food in the fridge looked old and out of date. He said "The man in the building is going to come and clean the place up tomorrow and that it will take him less than fifteen minutes!" Of particular concern to the psychiatrist was his chain smoking and setting some tissue paper alight in a wastebasket. The diagnosis of "senile squalor" was made and he was admitted to a psychiatric hospital.

After hospitalization, he was considered a "high level" patient, went to the hospital pub and liked watching T.V. He seemed kind to other patients and liked to talk to them. His only inappropriate behaviour was being verbal about woman's body parts; for instance he would say to nurses, "I like your ass." Neuropsychological examination showed surprisingly intact cognitive and executive function, but his scores were elevated on a mania scale indicating "expansive mood" and impulsive test performance. He tended to answer questions in greater detail than was necessary. Frontal lobe dementia was suspected and he was referred to our clinic.

When I first met him he was pleasant, talkative but somewhat rambling. He was dressed in a double-breasted suit complete with a bow tie. Far from appearing demented, he was well oriented in time, place and person. He knew recent history well, in fact, he knew more about international politics and the Balkan situation than most Canadians. For instance, he remembered President Bush was in Russia and was discussing nuclear treaties with Putin. He recalled his past medical history accurately, he did not think he should be institutionalized and resented the psychiatrist for calling him a "firebug". He blamed the fires and cigarette burns on his poor eyesight. He had a normal score on the Mini Mental State Examination (MMSE), forgetting only one memory item after distraction.

A year later he had declined and neuropsychological testing showed significant and diffuse cognitive change since hospitalization. The overwhelming behavioural abnormality and the preserved memory and visuospatial function at the onset and initial stages of his illness were more compatible with FTD than with Alzheimer's disease. Unfortunately, he died without post-mortem several years later.

Diogenes was the elderly Greek philosopher who vowed poverty, lived in a barrel and sought an honest man with his lamp in vain. His name became somewhat disrespectfully attached to senile squalor, known also as the "Diogenes Syndrome." The diagnosis is applied to individuals who end up living in a state of utter squalor, neglecting to clean or acceptably maintain their place or themselves. Family help or social assistance is often refused. They do not throw anything out, hoard scraps, and even hunt in the garbage of others even though they may have money. They may be surprisingly intact cognitively and capable of managing amidst large piles of paper, boxes, and an assortment of hoarded material including expired medicines and food. Their hoarding is often viewed as an exaggerated personality trait. They may have an obsessive-compulsive disorder (see discussion in Chapter 5) or delusions of poverty. Senile squalor or the Diogenes Syndrome usually occurs in individuals who live alone. Some of the elderly FTD patients may become homeless in an early stage of their illness, but they rarely have enough executive function or strength to live on the street beyond a certain age. The squalor of the younger homeless is often related to other mental illnesses, such as paranoid schizophrenia, alcohol or drug addiction.

Hoarding may be associated with extreme frugality or inability to spend money. Those who hoard and save to the extreme seemed to be obsessed with money and poverty, and lose their judgment concerning their resources. Ironically, although Gregory was diagnosed to have senile squalor by the geriatric psychiatrist, he was a spender and went through a large amount of money as he was sinking into squalor, just like Gwen, the other sexy senior. It seems those who spend impulsively and hoard at the same time are suffering from both disinhibited and obsessive behaviour. Impulsive spending and hoarding may appear together in FTD/Pick's disease. Compulsive shopping also involves excessive spending, but it may have different psychological dynamics from hoarding. When impulsive spending or compulsive shopping leads to financial problems, or shoplifting, the family urgently seeks help, with or without the law becoming involved.

Examples of impulsive behaviour and poor judgment in other patients.

...likes spending money...tips waitress before the bill...quit working on impulse when husband retired...bought a rabbit on impulse... makes comments without thinking...makes impulsive and irrelevant statements...spent a lot of money on his credit cards...wanted to ask a stranger to marry him...speaks without thinking...spends money impulsively...will make comments about people without

thinking first...bought another car on impulse...walks into the room and impulsively changes the channel...walks in front of bicycles and cars, does not look both ways...in the parking lot does not look, just drives out...took out $900 from the bank and when husband asked her why, she said she did not know ...gave large sums of money to a voluntary nursing association also a religious organization with the total coming to $15,000 on a modest pension income... she would take out several hundred dollars from her bank machine several days in a row...she spent $9,000 for six windows on an offer from strangers, even though her son-in-law is in construction and could have arranged it for a fraction of the cost...one of his hobbies is to go out shopping and come home with "bargains," but he seems to buy inappropriate amounts of these as well...she bought a $500 vacuum cleaner that she did not need...he acquired $800 worth of greeting cards and $4,000 worth of books...in a pet store wanted to buy anything soft and fuzzy... he bought another car without telling his wife, even though they can ill afford it...bought hockey cards instead of groceries...he became careless with his money, giving it away to church or charities several times a month, often on the telephone... she lost $5000 on an internet scam after she was notified she had won millions, and she still owes the bank...

Financial difficulties, impulsive spending and hoarding by a patient who may be otherwise rational and cognitively unimpaired as was the case with Gregory and Gwen leads to confrontation with families and caregivers. These patients may provide superficially plausible explanations for their spending. Their rationalization extends to other inappropriate behaviour. Gregory dismissed his car accidents and blamed his suspension of driving privileges, the cigarette burns and minor fires on visual problems. Patients with relatively intact cognition yet lacking insight argue with caregivers, or physicians justifying, or denying their actions. Physicians encountering these kinds of individuals, especially those who perform well on cognitive tests, wonder if the behaviours the caregivers are complaining about are just exaggerated eccentricity and may be reluctant to interfere. There is a considerable overlap between eccentricity and behavioural abnormality. In many instances of FTD/Pick's disease however, the caregivers have to go through major confrontation with the patients because of the serious consequences of personal neglect, poor judgment, financial irresponsibility, and social inappropriateness. Occasionally coworkers, police, or social agencies will initiate assessment.

Relatives at a distance from the patient may not fully appreciate the problems. Sometimes two sets of caregivers or relatives are pitted against each other in a battle for power of attorney or inheritance. A frequent pattern is the common-law wife or husband who has been taking care of the patient without formal arrangements and has to work out legal matters with the children who are not around the patient. These caregivers may be accused of acting for monetary gain by the other relatives. A recent example in the news was the fight over the estate of actor Charles Bronson of "Death Wish" fame, between his six children and his younger third wife who took care of him during his Alzheimer's disease. In his final days his children would not allow him to be taken off life support, even though his wish was to die at home. An even more recent example is the much publicized battle between the husband and parents of Terry Schiavo to keep her feeding tube in place. Her husband was also accused of monetary motivation. Wills and powers of attorney need to be complemented by advance directives about the level of health care in various conditions. These directives are called "living wills" and when provided by a person before the illness robs them of the ability to decide, they are very useful in avoiding later disputes.

Twelve

In Trouble with the Law
(Social Failure)

G ORDON WAS A 39 year old businessman, whose changes in personality and behaviour led to the break-up
of his business and family. He became socially inappropriate, disinhibited, and perseverative, made several
poor business decisions and borrowed heavily to cover
his losses, mainly from family members. Later he went
bankrupt and was charged with fraud. He was referred
for neurological investigation, complaining of word finding difficulty and forgetfulness, about two or three years
after the onset of his symptoms. His "forgetting" was
to a degree not a memory loss for events, but a catch-
word for a host of things such as inattention, neglect
and perseverative, repetitive behaviour. At that time, he
was still driving a car, picked up his children from school
and remained fully oriented. His family recalled several
repetitive, unnecessary and somewhat frantic telephone

calls at the beginning of his illness that were totally out of character. Later other instances of bizarre behaviour were recorded. For instance he asked for money from the examining physician, which undoubtedly speeded up his referral, more than any other symptom.

He came alone for the interview, because by then he was separated from his wife, and he did not bother asking anybody else. Not having a collateral history other than the referral note was a disadvantage, but I had seen his father and his uncle with a similar dementia 15 years before and was aware of the familial nature of his illness (see the chapter "A Wonderful Life.") Later I called his estranged wife, who seemed reluctant to talk about him, but she told me his personality changes, such as impulsivity and inconsideration, were evident probably before his social disinhibition became a problem.

On neurological examination he was cooperative but restless, standing up several times. He often changed topics and taking a history was exasperating, because of his tangentiality, perseveration, inattention, and inappropriate remarks. He seemed to have his own agenda. Instead of answering questions, he reiterated his concern over some of his symptoms already discussed and his current financial state. Often he would get up, leave the room, and walk around. When he returned, he was easily distractible and touched items in the room compulsively. He was oriented but did not seem to have the details of recent events and he had frequent word finding difficulty.

He also had some of the primitive reflexes suggesting the loss of the inhibitory influence of the frontal lobes. One of these is the so called "palmomental reflex": on scratching his palm, the muscles on his chin contracted involuntarily.

Now this can be an ambiguous sign in an elderly person, not necessarily abnormal, but in a 39 year old it is telltale evidence of disease. An electroencephalogram (EEG)[25] was normal, and MRI showed mainly left frontotemporal atrophy. Formal neuropsychological examination still indicated normal I.Q., visuospatial function, memory and calculation. However, poor organizational approach when copying a complex figure, many intrusions and a tendency to perseverate were considered characteristic of frontal lobe impairment. His attention, concentration, abstraction, and reasoning, the domains collectively called executive functions of the frontal lobes, were affected.

When he was caught stealing in shopping malls the police brought him for psychiatric assessment and after that he remained in the hospital, because of his continuing inappropriate behaviour. Eventually, he was transferred to a nursing home where he was alternately restless and listless, apathetic. He went around grabbing food, especially cookies, from the plates of others. Later he became mute and wheelchair-ridden. He died at the age of 45, eight years after the onset, choking on a cookie, much like his father years before. His brain on autopsy showed a variant of Pick's disease with ubiquitin positive, tau negative neuronal inclusions, the same post-mortem abnormalities as the "banana lady's" in Chapter 1 and more than half of FTD patients who come to autopsy. The family history included not only his father and uncle mentioned above, but also three aunts and later two of his sisters, indicating the dominant pattern of inheritance of illness (see the chapters "Sister Moria and Sister Act II").

---

25 Brain waves (electroencephalography) tend to be normal early on, in contrast to Alzheimer's disease where abnormal slow waves appear early.

The personality change and social inappropriateness combined with poor decision-making, planning and judgment lead
to job and marriage failure in many younger individuals with
FTD. The impairment of the now popularly called "executive
functions" such as judgment and planning can be the first sign,
but it is soon coupled with the personality changes and strange
behaviour, ending careers and social relationships. Shoplifting
is seen frequently in FTD and it may be mistakenly called
"kleptomania". It is probably more related to the compulsion to
touch or hoard, than to the compulsion to experience the thrill
of stealing as it is in psychiatrically defined kleptomania. Social
disinhibition, impulsivity, and lack of consideration of the consequences probably contribute equally, if not more in FTD.

Circumscribed, "true" kleptomania is a form of compulsion
that is usually seen as a life-long obsession beginning in younger
individuals. It is rarely done for monetary gain or the desire to
own or hoard like other forms of shoplifting. These individuals
(more recently a famous, young Hollywood actress appears to
be a celebrity example) take pleasure in the thrill of stealing, not
in possessing the items, which they often discard. Some persist,
despite being caught, and will resist treatment, because the act
of stealing is an actual "high" or "fix" for their underlying problems or neurosis. Another notorious case was that of a Canadian
politician caught stealing a diamond ring and got away with it,
blaming depression. He recently surfaced to run for office again
and lost, indicating the electorate is not all that gullible. Minor
forms of pilfering and the impulsive taking of things that do no
belong to them are more characteristic of FTD/Pick's patients.
Most of the time caregivers are aware of this behaviour and take

steps to prevent it. Younger patients who are on their own like Gordon are more likely to get into trouble.

Antisocial behaviour may lead into conflict with the law, but most of the time the strangeness of the associated behaviours becomes obvious to police, lawyers and other law enforcement officials. FTD patients may shoplift, but they do not commit robbery or serial murder as notorious sociopaths such as Baby Faced Nelson, Ted Bundy, or Karla Homolka. Older ones like Gregory are rarely charged and younger ones with odd behaviour or speech also end up in emergency departments and in psychiatric institutions. Antisocial personality, borderline personality disorder, or sociopathy are labels which may be used mistakenly for these individuals. Often relatives or concerned friends recognize the behaviours as being totally out of character and seek further medical assessment. Trouble with the law is the consequence of social disinhibition, poor judgment, impulsivity and lack of insight, which are new behaviours for these patients, not a life-long personality disorder.

Recently, it has been emphasized that patients who act as if they did not understand the consequence of their action, lack a "theory" of mind of other persons, or what "others would think."[26] To put it simply, they are consistently and outrageously inconsiderate. Patients with frontal lobe damage do not seem to learn from mistakes, punishment or reward, and make erroneous and inappropriate decisions for immediate rather than long term gain. Caregivers in our support group ask: *"How come he does not realize the consequences of his actions and what he says? He is not deaf or blind; he can hear himself*

---

26 It used to be called the "superego" imposed by social integration, culture specific rules, and education. This Freudian formulation of the impulsive, subconscious "Id", driven by basic instincts and appetites, but controlled and subjugated by the "superego" has fallen into disfavor and replaced by a number of other concepts, based on the experimental approaches of cognitive science.

*and see how people react with disbelief and rejection, why can't he
learn from his social mistakes and foul-ups?"* This is closely tied
to impulsivity and to what used to be called a lack of judgment,
the Freudian "id" overcoming the "superego". A similar lack of
consideration of others can be seen in sociopathic personality disorders and an extreme form is autism, where there is a
severe impairment or even absence of interpreting the reaction
of others, but these are life-long afflictions, not developing in
middle or late life.

Various experiments have been devised to measure impulsivity and judgment in decision making, such as the ability to
estimate risks and rewards in a card game for instance. The so-
called Iowa card game by Bechara and his associates uses decks
of cards with low rewards and low risks and high rewards, but
also high losses. Patients with frontal damage were unable to
inhibit their seeking of immediate high rewards even when
it became evident that they will lose big on the long run.
Functional brain imaging during these experiments suggested
the inner, centrally facing and lower (orbitofrontal) cortex of
the frontal lobes and their connections to the areas responsible
for emotions are important for decision making, and also form
the neural basis of moral behaviour.

Experiments with other cases of frontal damage indicate that
these patients do not lack social knowledge, or even the ability
to choose right from wrong, but they have a major disconnect
between the emotional experience and the social consequence
of certain behaviours. Mario Mendez and his colleagues have
carried out some of these experiments with FTD patients,
who managed the correct moral choice, but they differed from
normal controls or even Alzheimer patients when the choice
involved emotion and empathy. The biological significance

of the integration of frontal lobe circuits of social cognition with the "reptile brain" of visceral emotions is best understood through examples of frontal lobe injury, where failure of this integration leads to indifference, inability to plan and social failure.

The importance of emotional undertones in our daily experiences and the body changes accompanying these in order to learn from them has been coherently explained by Damasio in his book, "Descartes' Error". Emotions and the associated bodily changes signal the appropriateness and the social consequences of an action or a decision for the individual. When we encounter similar situations in the future, our reactions and the rational decisions deriving from them depend on our ability to experience these, and act upon them appropriately within the social context. Descartes defined the essence of being human as rationality or rational thinking "cogito ergo sum" (I think, therefore I am) but his error, according to Damasio, was the separation of body from the mind, rationality from the visceral, the gut reaction that guides the right choice based on accumulated experience, reinforced with emotions. A similar "gut reaction" was emphasized in the instant decision making process of "thinking without thinking", in the recent book entitled "Blink" by Malcolm Gladwell. Acting instinctively can be successful if based on experience, but can be disastrous if it uses wrong cues, prejudice or is driven by disconnected impulsivity such as in FTD patients.

Social intelligence, and its cognate notion of "emotional IQ", has become a prominent concept recently, competing for importance with general or instrumental intelligence, including mathematical, spatial and verbal cognition. Byrne and Whiten have described the successful social manipula-

tion and duplicity of monkeys and apes, which they likened
to what Machiavelli recommended for politicians 500 years
ago. According to the "Machiavellian ape" hypothesis, the
evolution of human intelligence has been driven by our
superior "mind-reading" skills. Higher-order intentionality,
for example: "I hope that she thinks what I want is reasonable..." etc., is central to the lives of advanced social beings.
This "theory of mind" (TOM) hypothesis of social intelligence has become a focus of research involving the frontotemporal connections of the brain. The unique development
of the human mind adapts to social problem solving, using
the selective advantages of empathy and the consideration
of what others think. It is this all-important function that
FTD/Pick patients lose.

The following are other examples of social inappropriateness or lack consideration for others or failure to realize the
consequences of one's actions:

> *...waving cars down the street...knocking on people's doors to
> ask for milk or use their washroom...singing and clapping in the
> hospital corridor...grabs a stranger and starts talking to them...
> makes loud remarks about somebody having nice legs...has rac-
> ist comments about people wearing a turban...calls people fat
> within their earshot...swears in public or in front of the fam-
> ily...was caught shoplifting, but a note from the specialist bailed
> her out...walks to the corner store in his underwear with a loosely
> tied housecoat...blowing his nose in his hands...yelling out dur-
> ing his daughter's wedding...borrowing items of clothes without
> returning them...swearing and making nasty, hurtful remarks
> to family...she harassed real estate agents and a court injunction
> forbade her to telephone them again...reaches into some stranger's*

bag of popcorn uninvited... drove sales clerks up the wall and berated them...dances to music in a public mall...sticking her tongue out at people...he would sit down at someone's table and take a section of the paper without asking...lying about damage to his car...locking up a union representative in her apartment...she gets very loud in stores...announces she has to go pee in company..."borrowed" books from a bookstore without paying for them...uses foul language in front of children and strangers...steals ornaments from other patients' rooms.

Experiments of risk taking, decision making such as the Iowa card game task mentioned above, or studies of moral judgments under carefully controlled conditions contribute to our understanding of some of the processes involved, but they are impractical as diagnostic tests in clinically impaired individuals who can not sit still long enough or focus on the task. They can not substitute for the diagnostic accuracy of careful listening to the caregivers' tales of woe. A behavioural inventory such as the one constructed in our laboratory helps to explore and elicit some of the common behaviours in FTD/Pick's systematically (Kertesz et al. 1977). This has been standardized in a population of FTD patients contrasted with AD and depressive cognitive impairment and was found to have high sensitivity and specificity for FTD. Some overlap in symptoms was found with Vascular Dementia (VD), probably because the small strokes causing VD are often in the white matter of the frontal lobes.

Thirteen

Sister Moria
(Inappropriate Jocularity)

Rachel had Power of Attorney for her brother Gordon (Chapter 12) and I first met her when we needed permission to obtain a blood sample for genetic studies (DNA) from him. By then, we knew that several other members of the family were affected, including her father (Chapter 14), aunt and uncle. She kept up a jocular, smart-alecky patter on that occasion and I suspected then that she too might have the disease. Rachel placed many phone calls to my office, which were initially interpreted as those of a concerned relative but my staff, fielding the calls, considered them inappropriate. A year later, at the age of 42, Rachel became my patient when she lost her job and her husband, Frank, sought help. Rachel agreed to see me only because she wanted to prove she was unaffected by the family disease. It was only after a considerable discussion back and forth that she accepted the appointment and then only on certain conditions. Her friend, Tracy, accompanied her, because Rachel said she did not trust her husband.

During that initial visit she was willing to talk about her brother, who was in a nursing home with end-stage FTD/ Pick's disease, but she denied there was anything wrong with herself. She acknowledged that her memory for faces was not as good as it once was, and felt that being unemployed had affected her emotionally. She added nonchalantly, "But I keep busy with the community." Her lack of insight and denial of anything amiss continued well into her illness, even when she eventually had to be institutionalized.

According to Frank, who was interviewed separately, the family became concerned about her taste in jokes, her uncertainty about how to carry out tasks and inattentiveness. During Thanksgiving dinner she broke into a song when everybody was sitting down to eat. Frank became very upset at that time, since this was similar to the behaviour her brother had shown at the onset of his illness. About a month later a severance letter came from where she was employed as a professional at middle management level. It stated, "Rachel's work skills were no longer aligned with what was required in her job." Frank suspected that Rachel had been let go because of her abnormal behaviour. She insisted this was not the case, that she was not ill and their lawyer decided not to pursue this matter because she told him not to. She was so keen to deny that anything was wrong, that she persuaded her lawyer to write a letter to me to forbid communicating about her to anyone. Over the following year several of her friends also voiced their concern about her change in behaviour, her uncertainty and repetitiveness.

Many of these changes were attributed to her reaction to her job loss or depression.

Her failure to recognize people whom she knew was interpreted as forgetfulness. She would attempt to cover up when confronted, saying, "You've changed your hair." She developed a strategy of approaching people she did not recognize, including strangers, and asking, "Where have I met you before?" Her children became very sensitive to this when she met their friends and expressed dread at the routine of "You're quite a bit taller. You have changed quite a bit." Her inability to recognize people seemed to be clearly worse than her memory for events, which was relatively spared.

In conversation, Rachel had only a few topics in which she was interested and repeatedly returned to these, regardless of anything the other person wanted to talk about. She also tended to ask the same question over and over again. This was initially interpreted as memory loss, but it became apparent that it was more of a preoccupation and perseveration with her particular agenda and ideas. Family and friends considered her constant questioning to be quite child-like. Rachel also used the telephone a lot. She could make up to six or seven calls a day to one person and eventually some people had put a block on their telephones to prevent her from contacting them.

Her constant flow of jokes, almost all of them risqué with sexual content and inappropriate for the occasion, was a major concern to her family and friends. She would approach a group of strange men seated around a table and say, "Have you heard about the ..." When confronted with her inappropriate joking she would say, "They asked me to tell them." Her fibbing and tattling particularly embarrassed her children. She would tell their little secrets in front of their friends. Her older son avoided being in company with her.

She became quite restless and could not sit still for long. If it was a group conversation, she interrupted people and interjected her comments. She introduced herself to strangers and spent some time around City Hall where she was well known, as her father was a former official. She would go to the mayor or members of the provincial parliament and offer her help. She answered many ads in the paper for jobs because she believed there was absolutely nothing wrong with her and once she had a job everything would be normal again. She even answered an ad for exotic dancers. One day she started to discuss what a prostitute makes! While shopping for clothes, she addressed a strange man, gesturing at her breasts saying, "I am a double D."

One of the earliest changes appeared to be a reduced depth of feeling. She related things that would justify anger or anxiety without any emotion. For instance, when talking about her brother, who was ill in a nursing home, she would say to a friend, "Come and see him. He is very cute." Her disinterest in anything, but herself was obvious when it came to world news, reading books, hobbies, or other people. For instance, not once during our interview did she ask me about the genetic testing which had been her major concern a year before and resulted in many phone calls to my office.

Her friend confirmed much of the above. She said Rachel could be fixated on a certain matter and call her everyday even when she was told a definite "no." When she was confronted with her illness she liked to play the

martyr. She often used the word "brain damaged" and
began telling other people her family considered her
"fat and brain damaged." Most of the time she remained
consistent about not admitting to the possibility of being
ill. Although she should have been aware that people
were moving away from her, she continued being superficially sweet to people and allowed negative treatment.
Occasionally she pouted like a child, especially when she
felt she was "left out" and made very childish comments
about it.

At our first formal encounter, Rachel appeared healthy,
well groomed and well nourished. She spoke clearly and
appropriately most of the time; however, when I asked her
to lie flat on her back during the neurological examination she said, "I can't be flat, I have big boobs." During
this examination I told her I was eliciting some reflexes. She
then said, "I will show you a reflex", and hugged me. During
serial subtraction she had to be cued, displaying a degree
of inattention, yet she was well oriented in time, place and
person. She remembered three objects, had no trouble
copying intersecting pentagons, but then proceeded drawing a picture of a dog that was unsolicited. Her Mini-Mental
Status Examination score was normal, 29/30. The so-called
frontal lobe tests, such as Wisconsin Card Sorting and Trail-
making, were not impaired.[27] MRI showed right temporal
and frontal shrinkage, but the left side was also beginning
to be affected (Fig. 5).

---

27 The failure of "frontal lobe" tests to show any abnormality in the face of definite behavioural
disturbances reflects an important dissociation from executive function and it underlines the
importance of quantitating behaviour and personality, in addition to the cognitive deficit. The
personality–behaviour disorder reflects orbitofrontal and right temporal involvement, while card
sorting and trail-making are dorsal frontal functions.

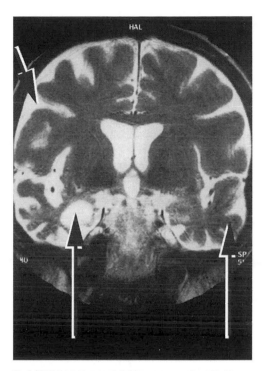

Fig 5: MRI bilateral temporal shrinkage worse on the right side
(2 arrows). Brain is dark. Fluid is white.
(Behavioral presentation)

At their request, I saw Rachel and her husband six months later. The purpose of this visit was apparently to resolve their "disagreement." Rachel wished to hear that she was perfectly all right and repeated her peculiar argument that she was checked out when she was 14 and was found healthy. I told her, in front of Frank, that I thought she was affected with significant problems, personality and behavioural changes. Even though she believed she was functioning normally at home, it was clear Frank had to organize the meals and other activities, and house cleaning had to be done by someone else. I was caught between her denial of illness and Frank's request for a disability certificate. I showed Rachel the significant frontotemporal atrophy on the MRI images, which is diagnostic of the disease. Finally she reluctantly agreed to apply for a disability pension and to return for a follow up examination the next summer.

Rachel arranged the next follow up visit herself with the agenda that she would hear from me that she was fine. She began the interview by saying, "I will hug you and kiss you if you give me a good verdict." This time Becky, her sister, came along for support and it was clear she was affected also. Becky's perspective was also that of denial of illness in Rachel, as well as in herself. She said there was nothing wrong with Rachel, that she was a marvellous cook and a marvellous driver, and she repeated this on several occasions.

By then, Rachel had floridly disinhibited, impulsive, and neglectful behaviour, which impaired her function as a homemaker and a mother. Uncooked food was left out to go bad. The pot roast the neighbours brought in was neglected and she did not come home in time to make dinner. They often had to eat out, or ordered food in. She continued tidying the house superficially and then she would disappear. The manager in a doughnut shop noticed she was going from table to table telling jokes. She danced to music in a public mall and twirled around with someone in a bear suit. Her boys did not want to go out to dinner with her because she sang to the waiters, ordered plum sauce with everything and nagged the waiters for more plum sauce. She developed a craving for sweets and drank numerous cups of tea with excessive amounts of sugar. She also ate a lot of chocolate and desserts, which became her main meal. She bought gum, candies and various other treats ostensibly for the boys, but she and Becky tended to eat them within the hour.

When her brother, Gordon, died of the same disease, she expressed sorrow in a superficial way at the funeral but lacked real emotional reaction. She would interfere with her son doing homework, insisting on talking to him and her husband had to remove her bodily. After that she accused him of beating her. Her driving became erratic. She made a lot of rolling stops, tailgated other cars, or pulled out too aggressively. Once she came too close to a truck, scraping it; another time she had a minor accident she did not tell about. She still drove independently and regularly to her sister's place 100 miles away. On one occasion she left the car engine racing in the idle; apparently the floor mat was wedged between the floor and the gas pedal and she was unable to figure out how to correct it. Her children abandoned the car in a panic and called their father who took her car keys away from her. This was more effective than taking her licence, which Frank thought she would likely ignore.

When Rachel returned she was overweight but physically healthy. As a prelude to demanding a clean bill of health she said, "I drive, talk, bake, and entertain. I am not fat or ugly." She would say one moment, "My husband wants to have me institutionalized," and when he denied this she turned to him singing, "I love you, I love you, I will never leave you," then turning to me, "I will pay you a million dollars if you tell me I am fine." She got up during the interview and walked around the room. When I told her she was still functioning well in some respects she said, "Oh great! I am going to kiss you. Please also tell Frank I am a wonderful woman. I am divine". In my waiting room, she burst into a song and a jig while Becky clapped and banged with her feet rhythmically. During her MRI scan she created quite a stir in the Radiology Department. She walked into an office and told a dirty joke to the manager of the department, a total stranger to her, then made several accusing remarks about how they were going to talk about her brain behind her back.

Formal neuropsychological testing still showed average intelligence, although she was probably above average prior to her illness in view of her occupational history, and still had some remaining islands of superior abilities such as calculating quickly and a digit span (recall) of nine numbers. On the other hand, she failed the logical memory tests (recall of a paragraph length news story) probably due to early verbal impairment and attentional deficit rather than a true loss of episodic memory. Her visual memory quotient was 98, in contrast to her verbal memory of only 70.

Rachel became more stubborn and neglectful, and her restlessness and childish fibbing less tolerable. When she developed a boil on her neck she blamed her husband: "because he pushed me." An episode of severely inappropriate behaviour with her children was the final straw that led to institutionalization about five years after onset. She would join children on the trampoline and on one occasion when the kids were pushing each other off she took a knife out to them saying they may want to use it to settle their fight. This initiated the Children's Aid looking into the situation. First her friends formed a support group to look after her 24 hours a day, but soon she was admitted to a nursing home (as fate would have it, the same one in which her brother had died the year before).

On her last visit she came with her husband and her sister, Becky, who by then was also in the same institution. Rachel's older son, who had grown to be a serious, handsome 16-year old, came along as well. I was touched by his maturity. He seemed to be in the process of accepting his mother as a sick person, rather than an embarrassment. They visited with Rachel regularly. She still liked the routine of going to Tim Hortons for tea and cookies. She insisted on a certain ritual of having the iced tea hot and having the ice and cream separately with two sweeteners, and the cookies had to be oatmeal. She had a friend who had breakfast with her regularly. Rachel, however, did not interact too well on these visits. Irrelevant things preoccupied her and she did not seem interested in the person she was talking to. She would interrupt a visit in favour of one of her routines like having a shower. She often burst out into inappropriate laughter or made out of context, irrelevant remarks. The notes from the nursing home were shocking. There was an extraordinary episode of eating feces (coprophagia). Both sisters partook in this. They were also found in bed together.

In contrast to these horror stories of hyperorality and disinhibited behaviour, Rachel remained fully oriented and her speech was adequate for communication, when she wanted to speak. She knew her younger son was at camp and Mr. Chretien was the Prime Minister. She could not concentrate for very long however. When she was in the office, she picked up papers and pens, touching everything on the desk. She also paced up and down during the examination like her brother, Gordon, used to do. She burst out in a song, "I love you, I love you, it's true I do/ There is not a doctor like you./ You are better than a pet./ I love you around."

She had no insight and claimed there was nothing wrong. When I asked her what she was doing in the nursing home she said, "My husband put me there because of what you said about my condition." She then proceeded to give me a letter, ostensibly from her doctor, in her own handwriting. It said:

RE: Rachel

1. She is fine and well.

2. There is nothing wrong with her.

3. There is nothing she can't do.

The same things can be said about her sister Becky.

Dr. Jason Walker

I had her sign it to make sure it was in her handwriting. It illustrated her relatively retained ability to write, but her continuing lack of insight, poor judgment and childish disinhibition to create such a forgery.

One of Rachel's early and most enduring symptoms was her inappropriate jocularity or Moria. German neuropsychiatrists called it Witzelsucht. Literally translatable as a cataract or flood of jokes, it has become associated with frontal lobe disorders by clinicians such as Herman Oppenheim, who documented what he considered euphoria and garrulous speech specifically with orbitofrontal injury.[28] The word "Moria" (silliness, gallows humor) was used for inappropriate quipping and joking in English literature. German neurologists were instrumental in establishing the frontal lobe syndromes and these formulations have been reiterated numerous times. Karl

---

28 The base or undersurface of the frontal lobes lying on top of the orbit of the eyes

Kleist contrasted the orbitofrontal disinhibition syndrome to the cognitive and motor programming disorder due to damage to the dorsolateral portion of the frontal lobes. Later a third syndrome was added when lesions of the medial frontal lobes were observed to be associated with apathetic, abulic, akinetic (lack of spontaneous, activity, and mobility) symptoms. The frontal lobes have become linked to various psychiatric disorders, in particular depression, schizophrenia, borderline personality and obsessive/compulsive disorder. In addition to frontotemporal dementia, which is a degenerative disease, head injuries, tumours, strokes due to anterior cerebral artery occlusions or anterior communicating artery aneurysms, or multiple sclerosis can produce many various combinations of frontal lobe syndromes, depending on the location of the injury. Of all the psychiatric disorders, a manic patient would be most likely to have the tendency to excessive jocularity associated with combinatory thinking and intrusions of irrelevant and grandiose ideas into the stream of discourse usually laced with flippancy and humour. However, this tends to be socially more appropriate than in FTD patients and it is not associated with the same extent of disinhibition and language disturbance as it is in FTD. Furthermore, it is unusual to develop a manic disorder in middle age. However, pre-existing manic-depressive psychosis can re-emerge and it remains the most important differential diagnosis in the behavioural presentation of FTD, especially if a structural abnormality such as a brain tumor is excluded by neuroimaging, or if the typical focal atrophy is absent.

Rachel's inability to maintain conversation, going off on tangents and interrupting others, in other words violating the rules of effective communication was one of the earliest manifestations of her illness and for that matter, of the other affected members of her family and others with FTD. This is an impairment of an important component of language called "pragmatics", which is beyond syntax, phonology and semantics, which are affected in aphasic disturbances. Pragmatics is a systematic study of the give and take of communication, relevance, topic maintenance and contextual coherence, through discourse analysis. Pragmatic rules of language are often violated early in FTD, even though other aspects of language are not yet affected. The following are examples of disturbed conversation in FTD/Pick's, often the earliest manifestation:

...Sometimes he just ignored questions and kept talking about something else...She was circumstantial and concrete...He tended to answer questions in greater detail, than necessary... She was pleasant, talkative, but rambling...taking history was exasperating, because his tangentiality...She only had a few topics she was interested in, and repeatedly returned to these regardless of what the other person wanted to talk about...She asked the same questions over and over again...He had stereotypic, circumstantial thinking, and an inability to answer questions directly...She had difficulty staying on the topic discussed, if other questions were asked... She used fillers or repetitive clichés...He was fixated on certain topics...She interrupted people and interjected her comments...He made a lot of out of context irrelevant remarks...She did not seem to know when to stop and perseverated with the same topics, the same jokes...The content of her conversation is corny, nonsensical or inappropriate...Sometimes he said things that were completely irrelevant to the questions asked...Her fluent and grammatically correct

speech consisted of frequently used clichés...She could not express herself coherently...

Rachel's social inappropriateness and the lack of emotional reactions were in striking contrast with her preserved cognition. This striking dissociation has intrigued neuroscientists and psychiatrists dealing with various afflictions of the frontal lobes since Harlow's 19th century description of the preserved memory and language in the face of altered social behaviour and personality defects of Phineas Gage (see Chapter 1). Other examples of social disinhibition in Rachel's case were the excessive telephone habit, accosting strangers, childish fibbing, tattling, making excuses when caught or confronted with unacceptable behaviour, and hypersexuality. Culturally specific social rules and habits are ingrained and rigidly reinforced by society. Transgression of these rules is as damaging, if not more so, than cognitive change to the family structure and to societal role. Work, requiring social interaction and communication, becomes impossible. Unfortunately, many individuals are affected in their prime when they lose their acquired social intelligence, while still retaining basic cognition in other modalities. When language and mobility are not affected, one of the manifestations of this is a curious flood of jokes, puns, inappropriate comments, garrulous speech, and derailed efforts to socialize.

Fourteen

Sister Act II
(Punning and Singing)

B ECKY, RACHEL'S SISTER, was quite similarly affected, although not when I first met her at a family conference about Gordon's illness and to take blood from her for genetic studies. Later she was seen in her hometown by another neurologist and eventually came to be seen at our clinic when she accompanied her sister for a visit. She behaved inappropriately, clapping and singing in the corridor waiting for her sister. They were both scheduled for detailed neuropsychological testing around that time. These tests were difficult to carry out because both were distractible and could not persist with the tasks. Their silly jocularity, garrulousness, stereotypic routines and disinhibited acting seemed to feed off one another. In contrast, quite a few cognitive processes, such as language, orientation, and past memory, were still relatively intact in both sisters.

Becky's illness began around the same age as her older sister's, in the early 40's and her behaviour gradually deteriorated closely following the pattern of her sister and her brother. Her boyfriend left her after she was let go from her office job. She neglected her housekeeping as well as herself. She was admitted to the nursing home where her sister was staying because she was waving cars down in the street, asked strangers for money (just like her brother), and resisted assistance at home, not eating the meals that were brought in, but living on cookies and raisins.

On examination about three years after the onset of obvious symptoms, she appeared overweight, but physically well. Much of her conversation was centered on the fact that she was well and she wanted to have documentation to that effect, closely paralleling her sister's behaviour and lack of insight. She tended to take over the conversation regardless of what the other person was saying. Although her output was perseverative, she had difficulty staying on the topic discussed, if other questions were asked. The following is a verbatim exchange to illustrate:

Examiner: What do you do all day at Sunningdale?

B: I do volunteer work, aha...At Sunningdale they are very pleased too. I am a former Air Canada volunteer.[29] Yes, aha. Both of us had scans voluntarily. Our dear aunt had the illness but not the scans. Older women have abnormal scans and that means nothing.

E: Why did you go to Sunningdale?

B: Because my sister is there. We did not realize Gordon

---

29 This is a semantic paraphasia, one of the early manifestations of her language disturbance or semantic dementia. She was an employee of Air Canada, but at this time she pretended she was volunteering at Sunningdale (in order to preserve confidentiality, these are not her real places of employment or institutionalization).

was so ill, because I gave him a lot of money. My brother-in-law had us hospitalized at Sunningdale. I lost so much money because of Gordon. I needed a job. I am still job searching, but I am over-qualified.

E: Who has your Power of Attorney?

B: My cousin, Lucy. Yes. Okay...My POA has access to my accounts. She initiated my move. I share a room with three older people but they snore and cough. They won't let me out. Both Rachel and I will require documentation that I am fine.

E: Do you have any problems?

B: I don't trust my brother-in-law at all. He is not supportive at all. He has thrown out much of the furniture. I do not have friends in… A lot of people have moved. I have my friends in… I trained a lot of people. Do you know my second name?

E: Yes.

B: Harvey Fagan, my father, was very well educated, you know. I went to York University. My sister to U of T. Yes. Aha. I stayed with Air Canada for a long time. One customer called me "Pagan." I was a reservation trainer and people asked me, "Are you related to Harvey Fagan?" I am responsible for his talents. I have his genes. Do you know Air Canada Centre?

E: Yes.

B: There was a man working there by the name of Murray Makin, a very nice man, a white haired man. I have a name theory, as you know my name is Becky Fagan. I could have married Murray Makin and then I would be Becky Fagan-Makin. Had he died I could have married a man named Bacon, who also worked there and I would have been called Becky Fagan-Makin-Bacon. On that note you are not mistaken, even though you know I am a Jewish woman (followed by a hearty chuckle).[30]

When Becky was sitting waiting to have blood drawn, her sister Rachel wandered into the room, smiled at Becky and said, "Do I know you?" Becky replied in a singsong: "I know you, I know you, you're my sister, Rachel Sue, Rachel Sue, I love you, I love you, my sister Rachel Sue." Then they smiled at each other and kissed on the lips. Then Rachel patted Becky on the head and said "good doggy".

The nursing home records documented pages and pages of severe behavioural abnormalities. She was at times agitated and unable to stay still, rattling and pushing about her cutlery causing a constant noise. She seemed to have a short attention span, playing the piano for a few minutes, attending pub night for a short time, and then wandering around asking for cookies. The notes documented fighting between Rachel and Becky, usually instigated by Rachel, but they also climbed into each other's beds. Then there was the unbelievable episode of coprophagia (eating of excrement) mentioned in the previous chapter. She became less mobile, had increasing difficulty with swallowing, and died recently. Her cousin, who had her Power of Attorney agreed to a postmortem examination of her brain.

Becky also had severe bilateral temporal atrophy, which was similar to the rest of the affected family members. The microscopic examination showed the same pathology as Gordon's, the so-called "motor neurone type of inclusions" (clumps of abnormal protein) in the same location and appearance as Pick bodies.

---

30 Compulsive rhyming, repetition and clang associations have been described in manic and schizophrenic illness as well.

The high penetrance of inherited illness in this family is deeply disturbing. It corresponds to a Mendelian dominant pattern affecting each generation of both sexes. One set of her cousins do not seem affected, although their mother, Becky's aunt was. I met them personally without formal assessment. They are stoical and hopeful as they approach and some of them pass the critical age of onset in the family. Their anxiety is reasonably contained but one can only imagine the emotional burden of this threat hanging over their heads like the sword of Damocles. The questions facing them are daunting. What does the future bring for my family? Are my children going to be affected? The prognosis of the illness itself is grim. The average duration from diagnosis to death in this family is between seven and ten years. Many of them, where records exist, died when they choked on food. There is a possibility of motor neuron disease (Lou Gehrig's disease) developing at the end of their illness (see next chapter), but other movement disorders, particularly PSP/CBD can also cause swallowing problems. In another branch of the family, a cousin presented with PSP, one of the motor varieties of Pick complex, as well as the behavioural syndrome.

Since our publication of the clinical pattern and the genetic studies of this family (Kertesz et al. 2000), significant numbers of similar families have come to light with autosomal dominant inheritance with the same histochemistry[31]. Autosomal dominant transmission often means each individual has a 50% chance of developing the illness if one of the parents has it (there are exceptions with incomplete

---

31 Histochemistry is the staining of biological, in this case, postmortem tissues with a variety of chemicals, often used for diagnosis and research into the nature of a disease.

penetrance). Only in about 10% of the families with familial FTD/Pick's disease, is a mutation of the tau protein detectable. We are continuing to look for other chromosomal locations and mutations. (See the biology and diagnosis chapter for up to date information on the genetics and the epidemiology of the disease).

Very recently a couple papers appeared showing mutations on the progranulin gene, which is also on chromosome 17 (Baker et al. 2006). This is an extraordinary coincidence and it could solve the mystery of the tau negative families like this one. So far no mutations were found in this family, and therefore predictive testing of yet unaffected individuals is not possible. Such testing is expensive, not available routinely and it is also fraught with emotional and social hazards. Some family members when faced with this kind of family background do not want to know if they are affected and will develop the illness later, but others are eager to find out. They may do it for their children or for the purpose of planning, marriage, establishing wills, etc. On the other hand, knowing the certainty of the future development of such an illness could result in major emotional and social breakdown prematurely. Specialized genetic services may use psychologists or psychiatric counseling in an attempt to prevent that.

Both Becky and Rachel reached a stage of childish, bizarre, disinhibited behaviour, characterized by jokes, puns, pranks, food fads, and utilization behaviour extending to coprophagia much like in the Kluver-Bucy experimental primates described in Chapter 2. Treatment for the time being is not specific but SSRI antidepressants, Trazodone, and neuroleptics are used for restlessness and compulsive behaviour. Insitutionalization takes place when caregivers or society (occasionally the police) cannot cope or keep the patients integrated in their former environment. Becky never married and her next of kin was Rachel, so much of the burden of her care fell on Frank and her cousin Lucy, who handled it with skill and compassion. For more about special caregiver's burden and means of managing the problems read Chapters 22.

Fifteen

A Wonderful Life
(Pyramidal Symptoms)

MOTOR NEURONE DISEASE or Amyotrophic Lateral Sclerosis (ALS) is best known in North America as Lou Gherig's disease after the popular ballplayer who gave it a human face when his career and life were ended by this rapidly progressive neurological condition. Who could forget Gary Cooper, as Lou Gherig, giving his farewell speech in the biopic movie "The Pride of the Yankees". Until recently ALS was considered a pure motor disorder and its new histological marker, the ubiquitin stained neuronal inclusion, restricted to the spinal cord and cortical motor neurons. Both of these assumptions turned out to be incorrect. First sporadically, then in a series of patients, investigators, particularly in Japan, described dementia with ALS, and later the typical inclusions turned up in the frontal and temporal lobe association cortex in more than half of the FTD/Pick's patients. Despite the common occurrence of this histological variety, only few of the FTD patients will have typical ALS and a few more will have some signs without the full blown disease, and many more the swallowing difficulty and choking at the end of their illness. The clinical signs of damage to the motor system appeared together with the behavioural disorder of FTD in the following story:

Harvey, a successful professional, businessman and later a politician, developed inappropriate speech and behaviour and stopped working at the age of 45 because of "depression," excessive appetite, and a speech disturbance that was initially described as slurred speech. The family thought "something was wrong", when he was only 38! He developed a dreadful sense of insecurity and inadequacy. There was childish behaviour and progressive personality change with impaired memory. He was investigated at a famous neurological institute seven years after onset. The report described him as having "stereotypic, tangential, and circumstantial thinking and a particular inability to answer questions directly." His IQ was still normal despite the behavioural disturbances. Pneumoencephalography, a standard neuroradiological investigation before CT or MRI (see Chapter 4 for description) showed atrophy that was considered maximum in the left temporal region. Despite the asymmetry, the diagnosis of Alzheimer's disease was made.

After his admission to a psychiatric hospital nine years after onset, he was observed to be wandering, taking drinks from other people, and interrupting others' conversation. When I examined him, he was well nourished and cooperative but his speech was difficult to understand because of slurring, continuing repetition of questions and perseveration of words like, "wonderful, wonderful, wonderful". He had a grin, inappropriate for the occasion, slow responses and after initial attempts he gave up on most, including the simplest motor tasks (motor impersistence). Unlike Alzheimer patients, he was oriented in time, place and person. His reading aloud and repetition were much better than his spontaneous speech. He was unkempt and neglected his clothing. The palmomental reflexes[32] were present bilaterally, the tendon reflexes were hyperactive, his left toe was up-going[33] and he was noted to have bilateral ankle clonus (jerky contractions on stretching a muscle, indicating spasticity). These were characteristic "pyramidal" signs of involvement of the upper motor neurones as was his slurred speech.

Later his walking became stiff and unsteady and he was admitted to a nursing home. He could smile and utter words, but conversation was gone. He craved sweets, overate and gained much weight. Eventually he developed increasing difficulty swallowing and was placed on soft food. He died ten years after onset at the age of 48, choking on a cookie, just like his son, Gordon, would decades later.

Insidious onset of altered personality, indecisiveness, inappropriateness, apathy, initially interpreted as depression, then progressive, perseverative, stereotypic behaviour were typical of FTD. Later decreased speech, mutism, stiffness, pyramidal signs and swallowing difficulty due to motor neuron disease were superimposed. On autopsy, the spongy change in the cortex was characteristic of Pick complex, although at

---

32 A reflex associated with frontal lobe involvement.
33 A sign of the impairment of the pyramidal tract, the main motor nerve bundles. Named after the pyramid like structures in the lower brainstem.

that time it was interpreted as a "long duration spongiform encephalopathy with motor neuron disease". The family history of a brother, a sister, maternal grandmother, one aunt, and two cousins was positive for mental disease. Harvey's sister had autopsy with spongiform changes and was the key patient for the first publication of this family. At that time the authors (and I was one of them) thought it was a new variety of degenerative disease, resembling Creutzfeldt–Jacob disease because of the spongiform pathology. Three of his children became ill with a similar disease (see the previous three chapters) and two died, showing the same histology of ALS type inclusions in the cerebral cortex.

Harvey, like many other FTD patients and other affected members of his family, showed a great deal of verbal perseveration and repetitiousness. By the time I saw him, his repeating everything that was said to him sounded like an echo (echolalia). In earlier stages, the recurrent questioning, repeating certain phrases or returning to favourite topics are often interpreted by lay observers, or even professionals, as memory loss. Early Alzheimer patients often repeat the same questions about their environment, which appears unfamiliar, or events they were recently told about or experienced. Their memory failure forces them to ask repeated questions, because they treat all incoming information as novel. This may extend even to the recent appearance of their spouses who are suddenly treated as strangers. This is called the Capgras delusion, common in Alzheimer patients, but I have only seen it in late stage semantic dementia with visual agnosia and even then without the reduplication or the "delusion of doubles". FTD/Pick's disease patients, however, do not forget the same way as Alzheimer's, at least not initially, but

they repeat and perseverate with words, phrases and topics compulsively. These are similar to the compulsive routines or stereotypies of actions discussed in other chapters.
The perseverative repetition of ideas, sentences, clichés and
words is related to the inability to switch, to the "stickiness"
of thought processes, characteristic of frontal lobe damage.
Some other examples of verbal perseverations or "echolalia"
are illustrated in the following paragraph:

*...She would repeat stories tediously and always played
the same music on the piano...He repeated the word "Texas"
enthusiastically and laughed about it. "Texas" was an answer
to many questions...She had only a few topics she was interested
in, and repeatedly returned to these, regardless of what the other
person wanted to talk about...She tended to ask the same question over and over again...His speech consisted of continuing
repetition of questions and words like "wonderful , wonderful, wonderful"...His favourite word was "excellent" to everything....She developed catch words, such as "advantage", as in
"it is an advantage to do this or that" or "patch" to express the
plural of things, as in "a patch of birds"...often she would repeat
what was being said, like an echo...the repetitive questioning
reminded people of a small child...Finishes every sentence with
"honey"...He would repeat under his breath "pass the salt...pass
the salt...pass the salt"...he calls everything a "vehicle"(he was
a vehicle mechanic)...he has about five little speeches which are
the limit of his conversation...repeats "peek a boo" incessantly...
says "nice" to everything, appropriately or not.*

Relatively few patients (less than 10%) with FTD develop clinically obvious, rapidly progressing motor neuron disease, but
many, like Harvey have signs of pyramidal tract involvement

such as swallowing difficulty and hyperactive reflexes. When it is combined with wasting or atrophy of the muscles due to diseased spinal motor neurons (the lower motor neurons), the term "amyotrophic lateral sclerosis", translated as scarring of the outside (pyramidal bundle) with wasting, is used. Behavioural and speech disorders develop in sporadic ALS as well as in the ALS-Dementia-Parkinsonism complex of Guam decimating some villages in this Pacific island. The epidemiology of the disease, which seems to be dying out, suggests some environmental factor or heredity. Oliver Sacks has written a fascinating story about the possible toxicity of the Sago Palm, or Cycads, formerly a staple food in Guam and the history of how westernization affected the islanders ("The Island of the Colour Blind").

A recent article in the New Yorker explores the controversy over the theories of environmental toxicity causing many of the degenerative conditions. One of these connects the eating of the "flying foxes", large bats, with toxic concentration of cycads, before they became extinct in Guam (therefore explaining the disappearance of the disease), with the more widespread accumulation of possible neurotoxins causing PSP or ALS elsewhere. Most of the science behind these theories remains controversial, unproven and often a matter of belief rather than solid evidence. A good example is the theory, popular some time ago, that aluminum accumulation in the brain caused Alzheimer's disease. This in turn caused a lot of people to get rid of their aluminium pots and pans. The brain aluminium scare turned out to be unproven and nowadays almost no one talks about it.

Sixteen

The Jean Fetish and Bra Obsession (Stereotypic Routines)

THE HISTORY FROM ELLEN herself was patchy and inconsistent; her insight very limited. She did not seem
to know why her daughters had brought her to see me.
She sold her home after separating from her husband
and since then, she claimed, she had difficulty adjust-
ing. When I asked her what was wrong specifically, she
admitted she was telephoning people too often, but she
seemed to be reticent and confabulating about her living
arrangements, marriage and work. She told me she was
living with her husband again after moving in with her
daughter and son-in-law. In fact, he did not want to have
anything to do with her. She said she was still employed
(she was actually off work on disability). A psychiatrist,
who had been treating her for a while, did not think her
condition was psychiatric and referred her for neurocog-
nitive consultation.

The story from her daughters was a disturbing saga of indecisive, obsessive and socially inappropriate behaviour for about three years. She became disinterested in having her family for Sunday dinners and did not want to see her grandchildren. The family more or less stayed away, but they became aware of even more peculiar behaviour when she separated from her husband and attempted to sell her home. During that time she engaged numerous real estate agents, looked at many houses, made offers and did not go through with them. She kept telephoning people many times a day and one agent finally obtained a restraining order against her. She ran up "astronomical" phone bills, and her daughter took the phone off the hook to avoid her mother's calls.

At work, a nurse laid a charge of harassment against her, and she practically kidnapped a union representative and forcibly kept him in her apartment against his will. Apparently she made an appointment with him to meet at a coffee shop and then she drove him to her apartment where she locked the door. When her daughter Sarah called, she heard a tussle in the apartment as the man tried to speak to her on the phone. Ellen was heard saying to him, "You are going to stay here until you understand." Eventually her daughter gained access to the apartment by climbing across from the neighbour's balcony and rescued Ellen's prisoner.

Another time Ellen ran a red light, collided with another car and tore off her rear fender. She just tossed the fender in the back seat and drove home. When her daughter saw the car she called the police. While she was on the phone, Ellen was shouting, "Tell them it happened in a parking lot." Prior to that, she hit a car in a parking lot and she just paid them $500 for the car repair and the family only became aware of it when money was missing from her accounts.

After a month of living with her daughter Sarah and arguing incessantly, her irritability, inability to make any decisions and perseverative behaviour became intolerable and she moved in with her other daughter and her policeman son-in-law. They observed further strange, socially inappropriate behaviours. Although previously a modest, even prudish person, she often appeared naked or scantily dressed. She became obsessed with breasts and brassieres, cosmetics and creams and used up whole jars at once. She began to make rude remarks about strangers in public, calling people "fat" within earshot, telling a child in a neighborhood to "go and get your awful red hair coloured," yelling at kids in front of her house to go home or play somewhere else. She used swear words much more casually than before. Paradoxically, in addition to being apathetic and withdrawn, she was also restless and agitated, getting up from the table in the middle of the family meal.

She developed a sweet tooth, eating candy as though it were going out of style, chocolate, oranges, "jujubes", etc. At the same time she stopped eating ordinary food. She would pick up a chocolate bar and start to eat it in a store without paying for it. Repetitive "utilization" behaviours included touching crumbs on the floor, patting children's heads, taking things from her daughter and at first trying to say they were hers and later admitting she took them, and making light of it. In the preceding two years she had developed soiling and urinary incontinence. This was investigated and was attributed to a rectal pouch but she refused to have surgery for it.

She liked shopping and she would hoard certain types

of clothes. As her daughter expressed it, she developed a "fetish" for jeans. On one occasion she had her sister-in-law take her jean jacket off so she could try it on, and then she would not give it back to her. Her most recent obsession was with jean overalls. She also bought a great number of brassieres and drove the sales clerks up the wall by demanding certain sizes and then changing her mind and returning the items. After buying clothes she often put them away, because she did not want to dirty them. She had been rude to sales clerks for several years. One day at a check out counter she wanted extra shopping bags and when the sales clerk refused, she started shouting, saying she had spent thousands of dollars in the store and she was going on a cruise, etc. When she was being served in a shop, she would tell a sales clerk that she did not know what she was doing and she would prefer to be served by someone else, without any apparent reason. Later she said to her daughter that the sales clerk was blonde and therefore could not be competent. She walked out of a video store apparently setting off an alarm (they were not sure how that was resolved).

One day she ordered a pizza from Domino's, which came with ten chicken wings. She liked the chicken wings so much that she called them saying they only sent nine and raised such a fuss that they sent 20 more. After she finished eating those, she wanted to call them again. Her daughter had to take the phone away from her. She fought with her five-year-old granddaughter over the T.V. remote. She wanted to watch "The Young and the Restless" while the little one was watching cartoons. She still insisted on wiping her and washing her hands as if she were a toddler and this created so much friction that the child told her that her brain was "not working right." Her other granddaughters, ages nine and eleven, were afraid to bring other children to their home when she was visiting.

She began to have increasing difficulty using gadgets or setting a digital clock, or new appliances. She could not use telephones she was unfamiliar with. She also neglected her appearance. She refused to shower and the family had to take her in there and turn the taps on for her because she was unable to organize herself. When they went out to eat, she always ordered whatever the others had. She had trouble deciding which chair to sit in and tried four different ones. She began putting too much paper in the toilet. One day this caused an overflow and she did not seem to know what to do, just stood there with water flooding the bathroom. Her daughter became aware of this when water started to drip from the ceiling to the floor below.

For a long time she refused to have any medical assessment and insisted there was nothing wrong with her. Eventually the family pressured her to see a psychiatrist. The diagnosis of depression and obsessive-compulsive disorder was made initially. Later psychiatric evaluation did not show evidence of sustained depression, and although she was vague and slow to respond at times, her MMSE was 28/30 and her clock drawing was normal.[34] A neuropsychologist assessed her but it took numerous phone calls to orchestrate an appointment. She refused to continue several times but paradoxically she was overly persistent or perseverative on some tasks. Her responses were concrete and poorly organized, and she

34 Drawing a clock, placing in the numbers and setting the hands has long been a quick "bedside" test of visuospatial function. Recently, it has become a popular test screening for dementia complimentary to the Mini Mental State Examination (MMSE). It can be impaired because of loss of drawing ability or loss of language skills or problems of spatial organization or loss of executive function.

had impaired ability to sort, to maintain a set and to change strategy. On the other hand, her overall intellectual function, visuospatial reasoning, drawing and memory were within normal limits. The clinical interpretation was impairment of "executive function" compatible with frontal lobe dementia. She had a CAT scan with enhancement, which was considered normal. The psychiatrist identified her behavioural disorder as "frontal lobe syndrome" based on personality changes and social and verbal inappropriateness.

The lack of interest in her hygiene, her excessive intake of sweets, her tendency to ask repetitive questions, and telephoning people up to 120 times in three days were all new behaviours for her. However, obsessive-compulsive cleanliness, difficulty deciding what to wear every day and a great deal of marital discord, including three separations from her husband, were considered long standing. She was said to have been suspicious throughout her life, and at the age of 25 was admitted to a mental hospital with depression. (She had threatened to throw her baby down the steps). According to her daughters, she was always eccentric, being obsessive about hygiene. She would use Lysol after visitors, told her children not to sit on concrete because they would "get piles" and was afraid of skin rashes. She was particularly phobic about lice. She also spent a lot of money buying the best clothes and cosmetics but her home was always clean and she was a loving and caring mother.

When I first met Ellen she was emotionally flat and lacked real insight, but was obsessed with the diagnosis and asked repeatedly whether she had frontal lobe disease or Pick's disease. Her memory was good and she was oriented in all spheres, yet she could not provide any detail of recent events, such as the war, or the recent school massacre and she was significantly impaired on tests of frontal lobe function.[35] Her IQ was average, but testing showed definite evidence of perseveration, disorganization, and inattention. Neuroimaging suggested very mild frontotemporal atrophy on MRI and on SPECT scanning.

She improved on mild tranquilizers, but she did not always take her medication, and the family could not handle her. First, she was admitted to a psychiatric hospital, then to a nursing home. She was kept on a closed floor and she seemed satisfied there. A letter she wrote indicated that she was nervous being outside. Nevertheless, she liked to go out shopping with her daughters and she still got into fights with them because of her socially inappropriate, childish and compulsive behaviour. When she wanted something, she did not like to be crossed. For instance, she wanted some jeans and when her daughter refused, she swore and spit at her.

Her telephone habit continued. She would make as many as 30 calls a day to her daughter's house, to former co-workers, to the nursing staff or relatives of the staff and eventually the phone had to be taken away from her. From her neighbour in the nursing home she had "borrowed" money, her slippers, and other items from her suitcase had also disappeared. Stool incontinence became a frequent problem and she did not seem to know how to clean herself. Most of the time she did not appear to have any insight into her condition..

---

35 These tests require attention, sequencing, mental flexibility, the ability to shift strategies, "working memory," and problem solving, all classified as "executive functions."

I saw her again after her hospitalization and she appeared quiet and subdued. She smiled a little when the small talk turned to shopping. When I mentioned her fighting with her daughter or telephoning, she just could not say why. Her behaviour during neuropsychological examination was that of inattention, perseveration and childish attempts to cheat. She left the examination to go to the bathroom several times.

When a repeat scan was arranged she refused to cooperate. Her daughters told me at Christmas she did not want to go home and when one of them insisted, she tried to choke her. Interaction with her grandchildren was limited and she made many inappropriate comments. She would say to one child, "You have pimples." Another child she would ask, "Do you really like your father?" She would say to Sarah, her daughter, "Your child is not as cute as your sister's." She would laugh at one of her granddaughters, who was just trying to learn to read and write and this child said to her, "Oh, grandmother, you are just like my sister."

Perseverating with the same routine, stereotypic, compulsive, repetitive behaviour (also called stereotypic behaviours or stereotypies) is common to the extent that it is diagnostic of this disease if they appear as a change in middle age. Although this symptom resembles obsessive-compulsive disease (OCD), the extent, the bizarre nature, lack of insight, antisocial characteristics, and the appearance of symptoms relatively late in life are features of Pick's/FTD. Repetitive telephoning, shopping at certain places and for certain items, checking of locks, doors and windows, clock watching, or the compulsion to have dinner, or some other activity at a certain time becomes a rigid ritual. Some of the compulsive behaviours reveal an obsession with health, drugs, pills, body phenomenon (elimination, sex, sleep) and money. Another manifestation is the compulsive ordering from magazines or catalogues, even the Internet. It is not unusual for these patients to get on "sucker lists" as they cannot resist sending in coupons or replying to special offers and advertisements. When caregivers attempt to modify these routines or persuade the individual to desist, often irritability, anger, even verbal and/or physical aggression is elicited in response.

FTD/Pick's patients are not aware and do not, as a rule, report obsessional thinking. They do not consider their compulsions as irrational or excessive and they are not distressed by it, like patients are with OCD. OCD typically begins in children and young adults, and these individuals are obsessed with thoughts of disease, germs, counting and touching and they typically carry out acts of hand washing and other rituals compulsively.[36] OCD patients have insight and although many spend their lives covering up, many seek help, as they are aware of the irrationality of their compulsions. Although there is a similarity between OCD and the obsessive behaviour and compulsive stereotypies of FTD/Pick's, the differences in age, awareness, extent and the nature of compulsions and associated behaviours are substantial.

Examples of stereotypic routines and perseverative compulsive behaviours in other patients:

...Stubbornly insists on doing the same things over and over again...focussed or overfocussed on one thing, such as picking up sticks in the yard...She kept telephoning people frequently and ran up a $300 phone bill a month...insisted on having ice

---

36 Jack Nicholson created a remarkable portrait of adult OCD in the movie "As Good As It Gets."

*tea hot, and having ice separately, and made a fuss if this ritual
was not followed...he drove to his favourite doughnut shop several times a day...sets out the dishes for three meals at a time,
cluttering the kitchen...goes to the legion routinely...insists on
being driven to the mall...she has an obsessive stubborn way
of doing things...developed a fixation on bright clothes, particularly with red colour...wants to go to the store every day...
checked his watch and coordinated it with his wife frequently
...she would practice adding and multiplying every day...she
would call the same people six or seven times a day... hunted for
missing objects compulsively...kept doing large jigsaw puzzles,
over 100 pieces...she would go around locking doors, windows,
and closing blinds...only showers twice a week at the YMCA
always after exercise...compulsively checks car doors and windows...he bought tooth paste and light bulbs repetitively...she
became obsessed with religion, reading chapters from the Bible
before going to church...all day he would be doing word search
games...he would fill out all forms that came in the mail...he
became obsessed about getting to his walking group on time...*

FTD/Pick's patients may have a psychiatric history preceding their dramatic change in behaviour. Some suggested this should be an exclusion from the diagnosis and
most clinicians consider only a change in behaviour as a
significant diagnostic feature. Ellen, for instance, had a
postpartum depression when she was 25 years old. She
was also described as being obsessive about cleanliness
and spending a lot of money on the best clothes and cosmetics all her life. It is possible that obsessive-compulsive
tendencies predispose, possibly by genetic linkage in some
individuals, to the development of FTD later on. Dr. Dan

Geschwind and his collagues have postulated this theory
in an interesting article (Geschwind et al. 2001). It is also
possible that Ellen had OCD that combined with a manic-
depressive psychosis in middle age and not FTD-Pick's,
but she has many other characteristics, particularly the lack
of insight and the asocial behaviour of the latter. So far
the combined neurological and psychiatric opinion favours
FTD. She exemplifies the overlap of symptoms between
FTD/Pick's disease and some other psychiatric conditions such as OCD and sociopathic personality disorder,
borderline personality, etc., which occasionally creates a
diagnostic dilemma.

Recent search for a brain based cause of sociopathic or borderline personality disorders led to the frontal lobes as well.
Several studies showed significantly smaller frontal lobes in
"Borderline Personality" disorder. This is called borderline,
because it seemed to straddle the border between schizophrenia and manic depressive disease. These patients are suffering
from a persistently unstable sense of the self, difficulty controlling anger, impaired impulse control, marked reactivity
of mood and frequent attempts at suicide. Parental neglect,
childhood abuse and head trauma, in addition to genetic predisposition are considered to play a role. Although there is
some overlap between these symptoms and those of FTD, it is
the remarkable change in middle age that distinguishes FTD.
Without a distinct change and definite deterioration the clinical diagnosis is uncertain.

Longitudinal follow-up examination and repeated neuroimaging suggests that Ellen is stable and she may even have
improved on an SSRI type of drug. The degree of improvement
appears to be greater than I have seen in other patients with

FTD, casting doubt on the diagnosis, although it may be a favourable response to the drug. Since the treatment is similar to OCD, namely using serotoninergic medications (SSRI's) or Trazodone (Lebert and Pasquier 1999), the diagnostic uncertainty causes no harm. Her family is hopeful that she does not have degenerative brain disease, only a severe, unusual psychiatric one, and I share their hope for better prognosis.

On the other hand, other families show some relief on hearing the diagnosis of an "organic brain disease" possibly because of the continuing stigma of psychiatric illness. Whether having a degenerative brain disorder is any more "legitimate" or preferable to a chronic personality disorder of a psychiatric category is a societal judgment which is undergoing a change. Some insurance companies pay compensation and expenses for one, but not the other. The organic and psychiatric distinction made in the past is gradually disappearing, and schizophrenia, manic–depressive psychosis and obsessive-compulsive disorders are also considered brain based, explicable by alterations of neurotransmitters or even structural changes.

Seventeen

Not Making Change
(Executive Impairment)

E XECUTIVE FUNCTION IS a relatively recent concept for a set of psychological constructs that used to be identified individually as attention, judgment, planning, sequencing, shifting, categorizing, handling conflict, making decisions, etc. Most of these have been associated with the frontal lobes of the brain, but widespread networks involving many other areas are implicated. The impairment of executive functions, such as poor judgment and inability to get organized for complex activity, can be the first sign of FTD, but it is soon coupled with the personality changes and strange behaviour, ending careers and social relationships. Executive functions are not only essential for executives or professionals, but people from all walks of life – farmers, carpenters, cashiers or housewives planning, organizing, and making decisions about what to do and how to do it. Almost all of our cognitive functions require some executive component, but certain performances requiring predominantly sequencing, planning, shifting sets, reasoning, and mental flexibility can be tested as representative of this overall domain. An essential component of the "executive" of the brain is "working memory", in other words, keeping in mind what went on immediately before and matching it to previous experiences, in order to decide upon appropriate action. Executive functions are impaired in many other neurological and psychiatric conditions, such as Alzheimer's disease or stroke, for example. Furthermore, they decline in normal aging. Even though their impairment is not specific, they are sensitive to early damage, and can be the first manifestation of FTD/Pick's.

Carol, a youthful, petite woman was originally seen for memory loss, but this seemed to be shorthand, a lay explanation for inattention and disorganization. Her trouble started when she was 46 years old, about a year and a half before her visit. She wrote several cheques to the wrong account and found various excuses for not paying attention. Shortly after, she began making mistakes at work as a cashier for a grocery chain. She could not focus and had trouble making change, something "she could do in her sleep before." Sometimes she would just freeze and not know what to do. She became panicky when her supervisor came around to check on her and she was then told she should take a couple of weeks off. However, she did not return to work because she was afraid to. Before that she was considered one of the best and fastest cashiers. She felt depressed and useless and she missed work.

Although she had plenty of time on her hands, her cooking became very monotonous. Chicken with mushrooms was a daily feature. She neglected to wash the mushrooms and could not organize the ingredients of the meal to appear all at once and it was a family joke that the dessert would be served before the main course. She would practice adding and multiplying obsessively, hoping to return to work and nagged her husband to check for mistakes or to show her how. She had difficulty with the access code on the telephone to her daughter's number and she could not program the VCR for recording. She got lost driving in strange places and when they went to a hotel she could not find her room. At Christmas she had trouble organizing the meal and the family had to take over. Her husband thought a lot of this was related to her confidence being shaken. She followed him around like a puppy and wanted to be with him all the time.

In addition to her inability to organize and accomplish tasks, personality changes appeared and she became distractible, irritable and argumentative. She withdrew herself socially and when visiting her daughter, rather than being interested in her new grandchild, she just wanted to go home. She showed poor judgment, talking to all the telemarketers instead of hanging up on them, even though her daughters tried to tell her not to. Everything took a long time; she hunted for an object obsessively when she could not find it instead of waiting for it to turn up, became very compulsive about shopping and could spend all day shopping for a white blouse. At the same time she did not clean the house the way she used to and she put several layers, up to six, on the bed including mattress covers and bed sheets in the wrong order. After washing, clothes were put away just in a bundle without being properly folded. She started eating with her hands, which she never used to do before and she put on some weight. Food was often over cooked and she left the kitchen in a mess, finding excuses when questioned.

The family history was ominous; her mother was in a nursing home for dementia for 13 years. Her symptoms included memory loss with relative retention of past events. She had a "strange personality" before she became definitely demented. She started having mannerisms in her 60-ies that were rather obsessive, such as closing the blinds and remaining in the house all day. She also neglected her personal cleanliness and later she could not take care of herself. Her maternal grandmother was also hospitalized with a diagnosis of a "schizophrenic illness." Apparently she was stuffing money in her socks and hoarding it. She isolated herself in the house and was saying irrelevant things.

Carol appeared anxious and had a little weep when we discussed her problem, but she denied being depressed or suicidal. Many areas of her cognition appeared affected by impaired executive function. She was unable to do serial 7's and made mistakes in spelling "world" backwards. She could not copy intersecting pentagons and made a mistake in the three-stage command. On a formal frontal behavioural inventory (FBI)(Kertesz et al. 1997) she scored 36, which was definitely in the range of frontal lobe dementia, although the neurospsychologist's report considered her to have anxiety-related, depressive "pseudodementia." The diagnosis of FTD/Pick's disease was supported by the CT scan, which showed frontotemporal atrophy. After considerable discussion, the family agreed to a trial of antidepressants.

Two months after starting her on Sertraline, an SSRI anti-depressant, her disinhibition and inattention continued to be a major problem, but her level of confidence seemed better. She appeared to have more initiative, although at times she said she was very tired. The family noted she became "huggy and kissy," and instead of just a glancing friendly kiss she tended to give long, wet kisses to her in-laws. She also intruded on others' personal space during a conversation. Although she mismatched her clothes, she seemed to be taking more care of her appearance and took more interest in friends and daily activities than before.

Unfortunately, some of her inappropriateness and argu-mentativeness continued. She let her dog go to a neigh-bour's garden and was very rude to the neighbour when she objected to the excrement in the flowerbed. She also showed some utilization behaviour, tended to touch every-thing, and pushed the microwave buttons randomly. Apart from taking the dog for a walk, she watched television all day. Sometimes she had trouble getting the right channel because it took two steps of punching the digits on the remote.

She talked inappropriately to strangers, approaching them with no obvious reason. At times the content of her conver-sation was nonsensical, corny, and inappropriate. She used fillers or repetitive clichés when she could not find something substantial to say. She did not seem to know when to stop and perseverated with the same topic, the same jokes and it was hard to get her off the same track. For instance, she men-tioned many times in a short period that she wanted to go to the "Blues Bar." Another favourite topic that kept recurring was, "how the baby played with her toes." She interrupted others during conversation and tended to come back with an inappropriate force, almost a paranoid response when somebody was making a remark which she misinterpreted.

Ordering food in a restaurant was difficult and embarrassing because she could not understand the ingredients and asked the waiter to repeat every single thing and explain it to her. After all that, she tended to order what her neighbour had ordered. She also developed a habit of splitting meals in restaurants even with relative strangers. She showed a curious inability to follow others when they got up to leave the restaurant or moved out after the theatre was over. She tended to stay in front of an elevator instead of getting out of the way. She had to be led "like a child" at times.

The story was somewhat different from Paul, her husband. He often covered up for her, obviously still much in love with her. He tended to be more forgiving than her daughters and did not mind spending more and more time caring for her. He would see the positive side of change; for instance, she was inattentive to her surroundings, but she also played less attention to things that used to upset her. Her daughters expressed concern about her driving because of her inattentiveness, but her husband did not think this was a problem and drove with her. She lost interest in driving a few months later and never asked for the car keys anymore, a relatively fortunate solution to the complex and vexing problem of driving incompetence in this illness.

When I next saw Carol, on her 50th birthday, her husband and daughters agreed there was definite deterioration. They were concerned about her inability to listen to what people said to her and her inability to recognize what was in front of her, even the most obvious things. When she was asked to pick up a bottle, she looked all over for it when it was right in front of her. Sometimes she did not seem to know what to do, standing in front of a car after she loaded it instead of getting in, or asking her daughter where her car was or confusing the front seat for the back. She did not seem to know what to do with her hands. When she was taken out to play with slot machines she did not know where to start even after she was shown. She had difficulty with almost all activities of daily living. She could not read the paper any-more and she did not understand what was on television.

On her next annual visit, she had deteriorated on lan-guage tasks and appeared aphasic, although she was still quite fluent. She made few paraphasic errors, saying "slag" instead of "flag." Her impaired comprehehension suggest-ed "semantic dementia". She could not repeat, obey com-mands, write a complete sentence, or copy a simple design. Her responses were perseverative and flippant; everything was "nice." She did not wait for the three words to be read before she attempted to repeat them. She did not under-stand some of the tasks such as the three stage commands and kept repeating part of it. Poor attention interfered with most tests including memory. On the neurological exami-nation she was very apractic (not only could she not follow verbal instructions, but she did not know what to do with objects, or how to imitate gestures), but her basic motor function was otherwise normal.

Further decline was noted a year later. Carol could not do anything for herself. She could not go to the bathroom alone, used dirty toilet paper to wipe her nose and could not clean herself. She was obsessed with her itchiness between her legs, underwear, and with certain dresses. She insisted on routines and kept perseverating, nagging her husband to do this and that. She said, "Hi" to strangers and stopped to talk to them. Her superficial conversation was initially normal enough that they would talk with her talking to her, but there was not much substance. She was put on tranquilizers for agitation, which seemed to help and she slept well.

On her fourth annual visit, Carol was still talkative and cooperative and had surprisingly good memory of her past visits here. Her fluent and grammatically intact speech consisted of frequently used clichés, but she could not express herself coherently. She remembered the September 11, 2001 events, but she really could not talk about it because of her severe word finding difficulty, wrong words, and frequent perseverations. She could not copy intersecting pentagons or write other than her name and this time she had a striking dressing apraxia, trying to get into the wrong sleeve of a sweater, inability to imitate movements or use objects (ideational apraxia).

Paul called a year later to say that Carol was in a nursing home, practically mute, incontinent, and reaching into her diapers to pick at feces. She was mostly in a wheelchair because she was falling easily. Her gait became shuffling, she leaned backward and to the right, and she could not look up or down, characteristic of progressive supranuclear palsy (PSP) when she was recently re-examined and had genetic testing done (see chapter on the Hero of Bolero). The results of the search for a tau mutation were negative, providing some relief to her daughters, but the uncertainty about their chances of inheriting her illness continues.

Carol presented with job failure and an inability to handle the complexities of her job even though these were relatively routine for her. Although this was initially thought to be related to anxiety and depression, as she was very upset about not being able to do her job, it now seems more likely a failure of executive function due to frontal lobe involvement, and her anxiety was probably secondary. Shortly after she lost her complex household skills, especially the sequential task of meal preparation.

Executive deficit is one of the earliest but also the least specific manifestation of FTD/Pick's. Occasionally it occurs at the very beginning of the illness and it is puzzling to encounter a younger individual who cannot cope with multitasking or the demands of a changing work environment. Without the behavioural and personality changes, the diagnosis of depression or "burn out" is commonly made. Indeed, depression can cause a great deal of executive dysfunction but the sadness, feelings of worthlessness, suicidal ideation, crying, and sleep disturbance are sufficiently distinctive. Executive deficit is also common in early Alzheimer's disease, in fact, it is a feature of just about any brain impairment due to stroke, head injury, encephalitis, or even "normal" aging. However, if it is slow, insidious and an isolated development in a younger individual, and brain tumor and other slowly progressive encephalopathy can be excluded by neuroimaging, FTD/Pick's becomes a top candidate for the diagnosis, to be confirmed by the subsequent development of behaviour and language disorder. This often takes one or even more yearly follow-up visits to confirm, as illustrated by Carol's story.

Carol's case is typical of FTD in many respects, but she also had curious visual difficulties, inability to scan or recognize complex situations. This suggested the possible diagnosis of other degenerative conditions such as the "posterior cortical atrophy" described by Frank Benson and his colleagues. These patients complain of not being able to see objects in front of them, or not being able to recognize what objects are for, or what to do with them. However, in Carol's case this was likely related to several other complex processes, underlying the recognition of the meaning of objects and situations. Her decreasing comprehension of words and her difficulty recognizing and naming objects, also labelled as "semantic dementia", was undoubtedly a contributing factor (see Chapter 5 "What is Steak?")

Another possible cause of her visual difficulties was the developing vertical gaze paralysis and lateral gaze deficit preventing her from scanning and seeing objects. Furthermore, she seemed to have no idea how to use simpler objects at times, which has been described in the literature under the rubric of "ideational apraxia", also a cardinal feature of the corticobasal degeneration syndrome (CBDs) discussed in previous chapters. This may have contributed to her initial job failure. Her social inappropriateness, rudeness, obsessions, stubbornness, indifference, personal neglect, and language loss came later. Carol's case illustrates how FTD may start with a combination of executive dysfunction and ideational apraxia closely followed by the personality and behaviour alteration, diminished language function in the form of semantic dementia and finally PSP/CBD, confirming that FTD/Pick's complex includes this movement and oculomotor disorder (see biology).

Eighteen

The Not So "Belle" Indifference (Lack of Concern and Insight)

NELSON USED TO BE A SHY and reserved accountant but he began making out of character remarks when he reached 65, wondering aloud how his daughter and son-in-law were having intercourse and pointing out a couple of birds chasing each other as having sex. He bought groceries they did not need and tried to make love to his wife during shopping. Sometimes he said things that were completely irrelevant to the questions asked. For example, his daughter would ask him if he would like to go to the Dairy Queen and he would say, "No, I can't dance." He bought $2,000 worth of windows that they did not need on a phone solicitation. Other examples of inappropriate behaviour included grabbing some strangers and starting to talk to them, or making loud remarks about somebody having fat legs. He was uncharacteristically aggressive with his dog, throwing things at him, and he also laughed without reason on several occasions.

His wife committed suicide (she had a depression, aggravated by her husband's significant personality changes), but he showed no emotion. As if nothing had happened, he resumed playing tennis and cross-country skiing. His indifference and extraordinary detachment shocked his daughters into realizing something was drastically wrong with him, despite his apparent physical good health, and they insisted on finding an answer.

When I met him about two years after the onset of his illness, he appeared well, but distant and disengaged. On the usual screening tests he was oriented, except for the date, which he remembered later. His cooperation was limited by restlessness as he walked out of the office several times. However, he could be persuaded to return without too much trouble and after several interruptions we managed to complete the examination. He was more remarkable for his preserved cognition, than for any loss. He would not have been considered demented by most clinicians.

His speech was normal in grammar and pronunciation, although he tended to be laconic and spoke in short sentences. His memory appeared intact, but his answers were glib and superficial. Nevertheless, he was able to tell me what he used to do in detail. He remembered recent events, such as the "fish war", although he would not tell me much about it until I asked him leading questions. He also knew that O.J. Simpson was on trial for the murder of his wife and another man, and he thought that he probably was guilty, although he could not explain to me why. He also told me he liked reading and when I asked him what he had read lately he said, "The Little Drummer Girl", by John Le Carre and told me the story was about terrorists and a girl who was "balling people." His sample of writing had no relationship to what I asked him about, but he wrote a full sentence without any spelling mistakes. The intersecting pentagons of the mini-mental examination were copied acceptably, although somewhat carelessly with crooked lines and he did double-digit divisions quickly in his head.

Magnetic resonance imaging (MRI) showed remarkably demarcated frontal lobe atrophy, more on the right side (Fig. 6). We lost track of him when he was admitted to a nursing home out of town. However, his daughter remembered our discussion about the importance of obtaining a pathological confirmation of the diagnosis and called us when he died approximately eight years after the onset of his illness.

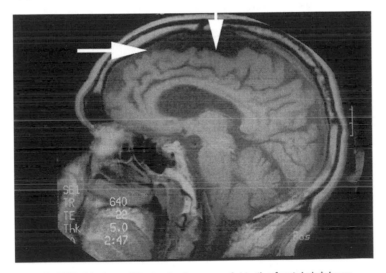

Fig. 6: MRI sideview of the brain. Arrows point to the frontal shrinkage. Back parts of the brain are normal. Brain is white. Fluid is black. (Behavioral presentation).

His brain showed severe frontotemporal atrophy with the gyri having a knife-edge appearance, thought to be a characteristic of the severe atrophy of Pick's disease. Swollen neurons (Pick cells) and numerous tau positive inclusions were found in the neurons and the glial cells with considerable subcortical involvement. The pathologist considered the histology as having features of both Pick's disease and corticobasal degeneration and thought it also resembled the hereditary tauopathies (see genetics). Sometimes the pathologists debate the exact variety, and although they may consider the typical instances distinct, the spectrum of pathological appearances overlaps sufficiently to consider them related. Some pathologists insist on emphasizing the differences, others take a more global view and view the varieties as a continuum of the same disease.

"La belle indifférence" used to be applied to patients blatantly indifferent to their disabilities such as paralysis or blindness. This was considered to be a sign of "hysteria", occurring often in young women without a physical illness. Nowadays such a sexist reference to the uterus has fallen out of favour, but the concept is still used in the context of conversion of an emotional disturbance into physical symptoms or as it is obscurely called "somatization" (soma=body). Such psychodynamic or Freudian explanations often invoked an underlying emotional trauma that was so unacceptable to the patient that the conflict was converted into paralysis or blindness, and to which the patient adopted this indifferent attitude.[37]

---

37 Indifference and detachment in the face of incomprehensible and unavoidable horrors are used as a literary device in the Nobel prize winning novel of Imre Kertesz "Fateless" where the young protagonist describes his concentration camp experiences with extraordinary objectivity and disengagement.

The bizarre nature of the behaviour change, when relatively isolated, may also prompt the diagnosis of hysteria in
FTD patients. This can also happen with primary progressive aphasia (see Chapter 4) when the severe loss of language
is not accompanied by any other cognitive deficits. One such
example was that of a nurse who continued working and taking care of her two children without much difficulty. Her isolated speech problem was considered "hysterical" by a whole
set of clinicians, who had seen her initially. It was Freud who
also described "hysterical mutism" as one of the manifestations
of neurosis, such as might happen to someone who finds it
unacceptable to talk about something. The Freudian explanation can hardly be applied to FTD patients, no matter how
peculiar and inexplicable their behaviour.

Denial of illness also has psychodynamic explanations, but
we know through a large body of evidence that it is strongly
associated with right hemisphere dysfunction, caused by focal
damage. It appears that FTD patients who are indifferent and
deny that anything is wrong also have significant right hemispheric involvement.

Indifference to paralysis is relatively common in acute
large right hemisphere strokes or brain tumors, when it
is associated with neglect of the left side and even denial
that anything is wrong, called anosognosia (the absence of
recognition of illness). This was first described by Joseph
Babinski, the famous French neurologist of Polish origin,
in conjunction with the neglect and denial of left hemiple-
gia. (His brother was equally if not more famous as a leading chef in Paris in the 19th century.) I have alluded to this
peculiar and bizarre, but relatively frequent occurrence in
discussing the "alien hand" in Chapter 7. A similar absence

of recognition of illness or lack of insight is almost universal in the behavioural presentation of FTD/Pick's patients,
although some will say superficially and rather glibly, "I have
Pick's disease" if they are told, without much understanding
of the implications. More commonly others insist there is
nothing the matter with them, or at the most say that they
are forgetful. However, the indifference displayed towards
the family or the plight of others is even more disturbing,
as in the case of Nelson, who not only did not grieve, but
hardly took notice of his wife's suicide, shocking the rest
of the family into realizing that although he was physically
and cognitively intact, there was something seriously wrong.
Other examples of indifference or disengagement in FTD
are listed here:

*...Ignores grandchildren...has no interest in family...dis-
missed her cousins in a few minutes when they paid a visit...
did not want to see the grandchildren...did not ask about his
wife's illness...ignored brother's death...she has reduced depth
of feeling...relates things that would justify anger or anxiety
without any emotion...apart from silence, did not react at his
wife's funeral...did not talk to family at Christmas...not interested in how his children are doing...she is emotionally flat, has
no reactions...stopped having the family for dinner...not interested in the baby, his new grandchild...inappropriate reaction
to sickness in the family... "forgot" his daughter was on the
psychiatric ward...did not seem interested in the person she was
talking to...never shed a tear when her mother died...instead of
going with his wife to her father's funeral, he said to her: "you
can go alone, you are a big girl now"...*

Indifference is a major and early component of FTD and it is often associated with apathy. FTD patients will rarely do things on their own and have to be asked, which may be labelled "aspontaneity". This is often combined with a lack of spontaneous conversation and decreased speech output (discussed as "logopenia" previously). Their disinterest in doing things ("amotivation") is included under the broad rubric of apathy. However, there is a notable difference between the apathy of Alzheimer's disease, depression, and FTD. Alzheimer patients are apathetic with declining cognition, some time after the onset, usually later rather than sooner. They can not remember to do things any more, therefore stop doing them.

Apathy, commonly an early symptom in FTD, is not associated with sadness, crying, sleep disturbance, impaired self-esteem and suicidal ideation, prevalent in depression, or with the severe memory loss characteristic of Alzheimer's disease. Patients with FTD may become jocular, garrulous, restless and continue to pursue stereotypic routines rather obsessively and their indifference to others and lack of motivation is distinct from the quiet, all pervasive apathy of depression. In many FTD/Pick's patients indifference, combined with social disinhibition and personal neglect, is the basis of strangeness perceived first by the family and then by others. Indifference and lack of emotional reactivity, combined with the lack of consideration of consequences of social and personal actions, lead to failure in social interaction.

John Fulton and C.F. Jacobsen were two physiologists at Yale who provided important experimental evidence about the function of the frontal lobes in controlling activity and aggression that led to the now abandoned frontal lobotomy for the surgical treatment of psychosis and severe anxiety. They observed that two of their chimpanzees Becky and Lucy, were particularly anxious, aggressive and "difficult", but became placid and easy to handle after bilateral partial removal of the frontal lobes. Egas Moniz, a Portuguese neurologist, who listened to their talk at the 1935 World Congress of Neurology, developed the procedure of frontal lobotomy for humans in association with Almeida Lima, his neurosurgical colleague, receiving the Nobel price for this controversial procedure.

The initial success of the operation was attributable to the extraordinary behavioural change in some of the patients, who had to be kept in closed wards before the operation, because of the potential harm to themselves or others. After surgery they became quiet and placid, yet retained their memory, intelligence and language. However it soon became evident that this change came at a high price: their personality changed, they became indifferent, amotivational, strange, like the character played by Jack Nicholson in "One Flew Over The Cuckoo's Nest".

There is a substantial amount of evidence from lesions in humans and functional activation experiments confirming the importance of the inside ("medial") surface of the frontal lobes, particularly the cingulate area responsible for motivation and activity levels (cingulum= belt, so called because it surrounds the structures underneath like a belt). The connection of this region with the orbitofrontal cortex (the frontal lobe above the eyes) and the temporal lobe, particularly the almond shaped gray matter called amygdala (almonds), forms a circuit of emotional regulation of activity, also relevant in depression and mania. The same neuronal system also regulates relations to others and society and forms our personality. This is why indifference and social inappropriateness are so often combined to form the personality change of FTD/Pick's disease.

Motivation is the mental process or behaviour directed towards action or purpose including impulse, desire, volition and striving. How behaviour is initiated, sustained, directed or stopped is greatly affected in a number of mental disorders, all of which share involvement of frontotemporal circuits of the brain. Disorders of diminished motivation occur not only in our FTD/Pick's patients and in depression, but also after head injury, which so often affects the frontal lobes, and in schizophrenia, where the negative symptoms are correlated with diminished metabolism of the frontal and temporal lobes, and even atrophy. Disorders of increased motivation also occur and some of the symptoms may coexist paradoxically by the FTD patients.

Mania has excessive and at times grandiose, goal directed behaviour, garrulousness and excessive pursuit of high risk, pleasurable activity. Temporal lobe epilepsy is at times associated with hyperreligiosity, hypergraphia, logorrhoea, excessive philosophizing and hypersexuality, also called the Geschwind-Gastaut syndrome. These are usually younger patients, and epilepsy is the underlying condition, but they resemble FTD in some respects. Various addictions are associated with craving, difficulty resisting impulse, sensitization and reinforcement, reproducible in animals not only with bananas and sweets, but also with damage to certain areas in the frontotemporal area that makes the animal return again and again for an electric shock.

Impulse disorders include the inability to stop action or a compulsion, such as checking, ordering, hand washing, clock watching, hoarding, eating, telephoning, roaming, buying and shoplifting; all observed at one time or other in FTD/ Pick's and in Obsessive- Compulsive disorder (OCD) both of which may share disruption in certain frontotemporal circuitry, and abnormality in neurotransmitters such as serotonin or dopamine. These complex interacting circuits act to appraise the reward value of environmental stimuli not just through cool logic but also through their emotional significance to the individual. The activation, intensity and direction of goal directed behaviour also depend on planning, sequencing and mental energy, part of the frontal executive, a concept discussed before.

Arousal and activity are also regulated by the basal ganglia and the extrapyramidal system which was discussed in connection with the disorders of mobility in FTD/Pick's resembling Parkinsonism. The connection is reciprocal: in Parkinson's disease compulsive traits and hypersexuality have been observed for years, and recently gambling addiction was noted, especially in those receiving the chemical adjuncts of Levodopa called dopamine agonists.

Nineteen

When the Parent Becomes the Child (Childishness)

S ALLY WOKE UP with a start when she heard somebody coming into the house. A glance at the alarm clock on her night table told her it was 4 am. She was in her late 20's and a sound sleeper, but lately she had been worried about her father and suspected it was him. She was used to Gary roaming the malls late into the night. This morning he walked home in the pitch dark, after he had taken a taxi to the mall, finding it closed.

Gary lost his wife when he was 52. At the time of her death, he appeared somewhat detached. Sally was concerned about this and also about his inattentiveness. He did not seem to be listening to what was being said and at times he appeared "confused", not knowing what he was supposed to do. He also became careless with his money, giving it away to a church and other charitable organizations several times a month, sometimes over the telephone.

Sally thought this was inappropriate considering he had retired young and was dependent on his pension. She took over the cooking and he needed to be reminded to help with the household chores. After the initial assessment, the diagnosis of "mild cognitive impairment"[38] was made. When he was reviewed a couple of years later, he had definitely deteriorated. He had had a couple of car accidents going through red lights and his licence had been withdrawn. He was put on Aricept, a cholinesterase inhibitor, because his inattentiveness suggested memory changes compatible with Alzheimer's disease. However, his young age of onset was considered unusual for this diagnosis.

Subsequently, his disinhibition and odd behaviour confirmed the suspicions about the nature of his illness. From being a rather shy person he became rather bold. At a care centre he would go to the fridge and help himself to someone else's food. Another time he followed the custodian up onto the roof. He joined a seniors' walking group, but after a while his walking turned into incessant roaming. When the group was finished for the day, he often stayed to continue roaming the mall and went home by taxi. He became obsessed about getting to his walking group on time and he became very upset if he could not go. He also developed strange eating habits. He would finish a chocolate cake if it was left in front of him, and always asked for seconds when they ate out. He did not seem to know when to stop. Once in the mall he reached over some stranger's shoulder to help himself to their popcorn (a scenario reminiscent of the TV show

---

38 "Mild cognitive impairment" is a mixed bag of diagnosis. Mostly patients have only memory change that does not reach the level arbitrarily set to diagnose Alzheimer's disease and continue to function independently. Many cross the boundary in time. Gary is an example of early FTD falling in this large, ill defined diagnostic category. Later on his behaviour was unmistakable.

"Candid Camera" in which actors, posing as insolent waiters, would dig into their customer's food, or take a swig from their drinks). He would scoop food on to his fork with his finger instead of using his knife. He held his cup out in the aisle at Swiss Chalet for a second fill of coffee and when he was not served right away, he would go to the serving station and help himself.

Strange routines, such as shaving and showering only on Thursdays and Sundays appeared without any obvious reason. He had to be reminded to shower at other times. He repeated questions, sounding like an echo: when his daughter asked him to pass the salt he would repeat under his breath, "pass the salt...pass the salt...pass the salt...pass the salt..." until Sally finally interrupted him. He also repeated phrases from the radio that he heard. He read books over and over again, yet he had trouble telling her what they were about. His language became impoverished, he did not speak spontaneously as much as he did before, and he had word finding difficulty.

His childish stubbornness and single-mindedness seemed like "tunnel vision" to Sally. When he wanted to do something he would not listen to reason. For instance, he threw a candy wrapper into a planter and after his daughter caught him, he acted like a child, attempting to do it again when she was not looking. One day he came home from the day program with a large bag of "Smarties" that he apparently had taken from somebody. Day care became one of his adopted routines and he particularly enjoyed dancing. He was impatient and impulsive. If he had to wait for a few minutes he would walk around rubbing his hands and clapping his thighs and then he might disappear. When Sally discussed buying a new car he insisted on buying it right there and then, and he wanted the impractical sports rally version rather than the station wagon she had in mind.

When he walked around the mall he would take napkins from each stall of the food court and bring them home. He unloaded them on the dresser and he used them to blow his nose. Sometimes he blew his nose in the food court incessantly, irritating people around him. He would collect pop cans on his walks, crush them, and stuff them in his pockets, ruining his jacket. He would sit down at a stranger's table and take a section of their paper without asking. He took a book from Sears without paying for it. Sally first considered he might have thought it was a catalogue but he hid it under his arm trying to sneak it home. When Sally said she would take it back he said, "Let me read it first." His more recent food obsession was for hot dogs and at the day care centre they were having trouble getting the sweets away from him.

On examination he had a vacuous smile and he echoed what was said to him, repeating instructions such as "Hold your hands out." He had a persistent blink on tapping his forehead (glabellar tap reflex) indicating a release from frontal cortical inhibition and a mild increase in muscle tone, or resistance, called "gegenhalten".[39] The Frontal Behavioural Inventory yielded a high score of 43. This was in contrast to the initial FBI score of 12, two years previously. His daughter now endorsed many symptoms such as impulsivity, restlessness, social inappropriateness, poor judgment, excessive jocularity, perseverations, obsessions, disorganization, personal neglect, concreteness, inflexibility, indifference,

---

39 An early neurological sign of frontal lobe damage is when the patients resist passive movements of the limb (gegenhalten = holding against in German, incorporated into neurological jargon).

aspontaneity, and apathy. He was put on Trazodone with a modest decrease in his restlessness.

Approximately five years after the onset of his illness his gait became stiff and shuffling. He could not use instruments such as a knife or fork and his meat had to be cut up for him. He stored food in his mouth like a chipmunk and needed verbal reminders to swallow. When he was in a strange environment, such as visiting his other daughter in Toronto, he developed urinary incontinence and bed-wetting, although most of the time Sally could avoid this by taking him regularly to the bathroom. He spent his day watching Disney movies, reading Harry Potter books, and attended a day program for Alzheimer's disease patients five times a week, where he was the youngest patient.

On follow up examination, Gary had a fixed grin and tended to be very echolalic, repeating everything like an echo. When he knew the answer to something, he produced an occasional full sentence. Most of the time he spoke very little, and then in a whisper. He had more Parkinsonism now, increasing rigidity; he walked with a bent posture at the waist, and tended to shuffle more. His balance was worse and he had fallen a few times. He also had trouble looking up (gaze paralysis). He was tried on levodopa[40] for his symptoms of Parkinsonism without significant benefits. His symptoms were compatible with progressive supranuclear palsy (see the "Hero of Bolero"). The last time I saw him, he was mute, wheel chair bound and could not look up or down.

Sally, who was his younger daughter, set aside her studies and career to take care of him, reversing the child-parent roles. Her dedication and uncomplaining good cheer made

---

40 Levodopa, also known under the trade name Sinemet.

it possible for Gary to remain at home longer, even though
to live with someone with FTD is a test of personal strength
and character. She is not alone in this, but she is the youngest
of the many dedicated caregivers in my practice. Eventually
Gary had to be admitted to a nursing home because of the
amount of care required due to his immobility and incontinence. A few years later he died and his autopsy showed
the ubiquitin positive inclusions that are typical with FTD,
but would be considered unusual for progressive supranuclear palsy indicating the relationship of PSP to FTD. Sally is
beginning to pick up the pieces of her life, and is taking an
active part in our Pick support group.

This reversal of roles occurs in Alzheimer's disease as well,
when adult children of a widowed or single parent have to
become caregivers at times to both disabled parents. The
"sandwich generation" is caught between the care of their parents and their own children. This sandwiching is particularly
evident in the younger FTD families where the children of the
caregivers are still at home. It is made particularly poignant
by the frequent development of childishness in FTD patients.
Other striking examples of childishness in FTD patients
overlap with excessive jocularity and obsessions:

*...flicking "surfing" the TV channels, watching Tarzan
movies...he did not know when to stop with his childish joking and teasing...he made noises – vroom, vroom like children playing with cars...at a restaurant he was beeping like
the Three Stooges...he denied doing things when caught in the
act...childish gesturing...boasting and fibbing like a child...
she fought with her five-year-old granddaughter for the TV*

remote...during examination she made childish attempts to cheat...singing during dinner...constantly asking questions in a childlike manner...pouted like a child, and complained about being left out...she would stomp off when her grandchildren made her cross and she was frequently telling on them...prancing, clowning during neurological examination...danced the polka around the house...twirled around with someone in a bear suit in the mall...he spends an inordinate time in a toy store playing with toys and he would not let go of a toy he bought for his grandson...patting her sister on the head and calling her "good doggy"...he was childish about getting the largest doughnut and pouted if he got a small one...he became more and more childlike and had a temper when he was told he could not do something...he would hide food under the sofa...in the supermarket he raced the cart around and threw a can to his wife to catch...shot at police cars and flying birds, etc. with his fingers, initiating the sound of a gun going off...peeking around the corner of the room, and sneaking around on her tiptoes like a child...he is like a three or four-year-old child now...

Some of the presenile FTD patients still have young children and some have grandchildren, who become very sensitized to the disinhibited, childish behaviour of a previously normal adult around them. Very young children may incorporate a childish grandmother in their games, but a comment from a six-year-old is revealing: "Oh, grandma, you are just like my sister". Others learn to avoid their company for fear of being embarrassed in public or in front of their friends. Caregiver counselling has to extend to this younger generation as well.

Twenty

Shirley Is Not Shirley Anymore (The Loss of Personhood)

A LTHOUGH SHIRLEY, IN her late 50's, was referred for memory loss, her husband described an illness which was quite different from Alzheimer's disease. Bernie, who was quiet, soft spoken, but articulate, expressed it succinctly: "Shirley is not Shirley anymore." Even though she continued working with computers and finances, she became restless, impatient, quickly angered and childish. She was not interested in people around her and appeared emotionally flat, even though she carried on with inappropriate, childish gesturing and jocularity. Although she had been a competent, take-charge type of person, often initiating and organizing activity, she had become quite dependent on her husband, unable to go after things that needed to be done. Her thinking became inflexible and concrete. She had trouble recognizing and comprehending situations. At a police roadblock for drunk drivers, she became panic stricken, because she could not understand what it was about and as a result, she had her driver's licence withdrawn. By the time she was referred, she had developed difficulty finding the right words to communicate. Of all her problems, she only admitted having difficulty recalling the names of people she should have known.

When she entered the office, she giggled excessively and made light of the examination. Impulsive responses, inattention and impersistence were evident. When she was asked to walk heel-to-toe, she started prancing about as if she were on a stage, moving her hands and hips sideways in a vaudeville wiggle. She did not pay attention to some of the questions, yet she appeared well oriented, remembered words even after distraction and did well on a serial subtraction task. She had no trouble recalling a recent European trip, remembering the dates and flights. In fact, she was travelling alone without any mishap. However, the friends she visited in England called her husband saying, "There was something different about Shirley." Her children also had been aware of this for at least three years prior to her being seen. Her MRI showed severe right temporal atrophy in keeping with her behavioural presentation (Fig.7).

Her previous perfectionism took an obsessive turn, yet there were signs of early personal neglect. Subsequent visits revealed her housework had become less meticulous and her cooking monotonous – she mainly used the microwave. She developed a liking for Tim Hortons, always ordering the "soup deal" and oatmeal raisin cookies, up to eight to ten a day. In a restaurant she only ordered chicken. Some of her childish behaviour upset her grandchildren. She would stomp off when they made her cross and she was frequently telling on them. When her husband was driving she urged him to go ahead before the intersection was clear.

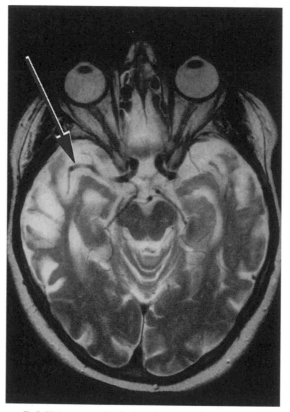

Fig. 7: Bilateral temporal shrinkage. Horizontal slice at the eye level. Arrow points to the right side which is more affected. (Behavioral presentation).

In addition to her food preferences, her table manners deteriorated. At Tim Hortons she would pick up her soup bowl and drink out of it. When told not to do it she would wait until her husband was not looking before starting again. She would lick her plate clean and she would stuff herself with her favourite foods. She would hoard dishcloths, shampoos, foot cream, toilet paper, on one occasion acquiring 120 rolls. Large amounts of frozen foods that had to be the same brand, always "President's Choice", filled their freezer. She became obsessed about clothes that were made of cotton and made in China and shopped for other cheap and tacky items.

Even though prior to her illness she had been socially most appropriate and pleasant, she became inattentive and hyperactive and in conversation interrupted others, making inappropriate remarks. Often she would repeat what was being said and this "echolalia" and perseveration were quite disturbing. At other times she would not reply to questions. Her husband brought me a letter that is reproduced here as an example of her disjointed sentences, quite in contrast to her previously excellent letter writing. The content shows preoccupation with shopping, malls, toffees, and chocolates and the grammatical errors reflect her progressive language disorder. In contrast, her writing is neat and her words are well formed (Fig. 8).

On her follow up visit it became evident she had trouble understanding some words. While reading a menu, she did not seem to understand what "veal" was. Similarly, she asked what was "power" or "electricity" (see the chapter, "What is Steak?"). She lost the meaning of words such as "robin, allergy, hay fever, pizza, chickenpox, lawns, waves, and tides," and she developed stereotypic expressions such as advantage, as "It is an advantage to do this or that." The other catch word was "patch" to express a number of items or pleural of items such as a "patch of birds."

anyway love the other reason I went for that walk on Saturday
I knew I'd love to quickly go to a Mall that is only about a 15
minute walk from ▓▓▓▓▓▓▓▓ as they have always had a
"British" shop in that Mall + I went to check they still had
all the Thorntons Toffees + other things. So of course when
I saw the Cadburys Double Decker chocolates I thought about
you love so I did get you two of them love + of course
you dont have to pay me for them love as you have always
been so kind + friendly to me when I've been at ▓▓▓▓▓▓
+ of course I will miss seeing you but I will always be
happy to occassionly be with you sometime + of course you
can also come to dinner with us sometime + come to a band
concert as well + as you know I do keep hoping that some
of the girls will miss me being at ▓▓▓▓▓▓ to help them + of
course I did tell Mike that I would be glad to come anytime to
help anyone even if it is just 1 day or a ½ day occassionaly at

Fig. 8: A letter from a previously highly literate woman which is now rambling, has paragrammatisms
and regularization errors in spelling and shows preoccupation with malls, shopping, and
chocolates. Names and the place where she worked are blacked out to preserve privacy.

Formal neuropsychological testing was difficult because
of her repetitive, perseverative behaviour and difficulty
focusing on tasks. Her concreteness and perseveration were
particularly evident on card sorting. Instead of describing a
picture she would read the copyright notice on the bottom of
the picture. She forgot the names of places she travelled to
such as Stonehenge in England but she remembered place
names that were close to her residence. On the behavioural
inventory, her husband endorsed disinhibition, perseveration, inflexibility, concreteness and indifference. Apparently
when her mother died she did not shed a tear.

Further on, her behaviour and personality change became
increasingly florid. Completely out of character, she went
up to strangers to tell them they should not wear high heel

shoes and she was hugging and kissing waitresses. On one of her walks she saw a couple having wedding pictures taken and she walked up to the bride and said, "Happy wedding." and kissed her. She often misunderstood what was going on and appeared angry. In a restaurant she would take food from other tables. She secretly took her husband's car and drove to Tim Hortons. She also took to spitting, mostly just saliva. She constantly wore the same clothes and neglected to shower. Bernie felt she would be horrified if she could realized how she looked now since she had always taken pride in her appearance.

Despite all this, she remained oriented, even regimented, and was always ready to go to bed at exactly 7:40 p.m. The morning before her appointment she would set out lunch and supper dishes for that day as well as breakfast dishes for the next day, even though the kitchen became very cluttered. She continued being active and walked a lot in a regimented fashion, sticking to a routine. When she was made to deviate from that she became very upset, even to the extent of being aggressive.

She improved somewhat on Prozac and Trazodone, which lessened some of her perseverative and compulsive behaviour, although she was still very bound by routine. Her speech became empty with very little relationship to the question asked and she seemed to understand less and less. She was echolalic, repeating everything that was said and perseverated with single words. She became incontinent of urine, later of stool, and began stuffing toilet paper in her underwear. She did not return for her fifth annual visit because she had been admitted to a psychiatric hospital after her incontinence became worse and her behaviour deteriorated. She died a few months later and her autopsy confirmed FTD/Pick complex with ubiquitin positive, MND type inclusions in the nerve cells.

Change in personality is a core feature of frontotemporal dementia. This often occurs to such an extent that caregivers and friends remark that their spouse or parent is a changed person, a stranger. Indifference, coldness, disengagement, apathy, lack of social interaction, disinhibited behaviour with bizarre compulsions, and perseverative, stereotypic actions all contribute to this impression. The personality change often takes the shape of rudeness, childishness, or lack of consideration. Early in the illness this may be couched in facetiousness or joking. However, it soon becomes apparent that what is said or done is not funny, not only "politically," but socially incorrect, inappropriate and unacceptable. Telling people off, impatience, cutting in lines, insulting strangers, berating service people, cutting off other drivers, swearing in public, or approaching strange children may result in social exclusion, retaliation, altercations, and even trouble with the law, such as loss of a driver's licence, and restriction of freedom, even institutionalization of an otherwise cognitively intact, relatively young individual.

This change in personal conduct combined with other changes in social behaviour has been interpreted as a "loss of self". A small number of patients who exhibited dramatic changes in personality and social values were found to have brain atrophy, which was more prominent in the right frontal lobe, giving rise to the claim that this is the region that is important to maintain the integrity of self (Miller, et al. 2001). One of these patients recognized the change in herself and

referred to the her new, neglectful, gluttonous self as somebody else, even giving herself a new name for the other personality.[41] In my experience, this degree of insight is unusual
for an FTD/Pick's patient and as a rule they do not recognize
the change in themselves. Others, observing epileptic patients
with right hemispheric focal electric discharges and stroke
patients with denial of their paralysed left arm (see discussion
about the "alien hand") also came to the conclusion that the
right hemisphere is dominant for maintaining a coherent, continuous, and unified sense of emotional and corporeal self.

Shirley also developed semantic problems, but in one significant respect differed from Rita in the chapter, "What is
Steak?" or Malcolm in "Houdini" because in Shirley's case,
the primary disturbances were the personality change and
inappropriate behaviour which were followed by the loss of
comprehension and meaning of things as a secondary phenomenon. In contrast, Rita, Malcolm (Houdini) and Jill, the artist, developed a semantic language disturbance first, followed
by a major behavioural problem in Malcolm and Jill, and a
relatively minor one in Rita. In others, such as Shirley, the
Fagan sisters and Carol, a similar semantic disorder appeared
only later in the illness. These cases illustrate that the emphasis
on the distinction reflected in the terminology such as frontotemporal dementia, frontal type, or in some articles the right
temporal variant, or semantic dementia, left temporal variant,
is artificial because these patients suffer from the same illness
and develop very similar behaviours eventually, or often at the
same time.

---

41 Multiple or split personalities most often have been described in the context of schizophrenia
in the past, although other psychiatric explanations, such as childhood trauma have been evoked
also, such as in the movie "The Three Faces of Eve" with Joanne Woodward and J. Lee Cobb as the
sympathetic and resourceful psychiatrist.

The emphasis can be on one or another clinical type depending on the time of observation, the interest of the examiner, or the anatomical structure that is seen affected on neuroimaging. When language disturbance occurs primarily, the left hemisphere is affected first and foremost. The left temporal lobe is predominantly atrophied in semantic dementia and the left frontotemporal area in the nonfluent type of PPA. When personality changes occur first, the orbitofrontal regions and the right temporal lobe appear primarily affected before the disease spreads to other parts of the brain.

Twenty-One

A Disease Lost and Found
(The History and Biology of FTD/
Pick Complex)

FRONTOTEMPORAL DEMENTIA IS a new name for Pick's disease. Pick's articles were clinical descriptions, similar to the ones you read in this book, with comments on the post-mortem appearance of the brain, aimed to show that mental changes such as aphasia and deterioration of behaviour could be related to focal atrophy of the cerebral cortex (Pick 1892, 1902, 1904). The basic anatomy and biology of neurodegeneration were explored with the help of the technological advances of fixation and staining of the brain tissue and cells with silver compounds and other dyes. Around the turn of the 19th century several laboratories discovered senile plaques, which later became the hallmark of Alzheimer's disease. Alzheimer used the silver stain and discovered the flame shaped neurofibrillary tangles and the senile plaques, which later were found to have amyloid, a form of denatured protein, in their core. He also found the round inclusions, "silver bullets," in cases of focal degeneration (Alzheimer 1911). The inclusions were named Pick bodies to honour Pick's description of focal, circumscribed atrophy (Onari & Spatz 1926). Later these inclusions were found to contain abnormally phosphorylated tau protein, similar to the twisted tangles of Alzheimer's disease (AD), but this discovery had to wait another 80 years for the development of protein chemistry and molecular biology.

Other distinctive features of the postmortem histology of Pick's disease (later FTD) were the abnormally large Pick cells, also called ballooned neurons, that are pale and achromatic (do not stain) and the spongiform change (holes like in a sponge, where tissue disappeared) in the superficial layer of the cortex. There is loss of neurons, the communicating network, and proliferation of glia (the glia are the supporting cells of the brain tissue which also respond to brain insult as well as providing other important metabolic and cleanup functions beyond their support role.) Although Onari and Spatz tried to emphasize these other features and in fact said that Pick bodies were not necessary for the diagnosis, the distinctiveness of these structures made them the defining feature for Pick's disease.

Why then has such a unique and far from rare disease become almost unknown in recent times and why to this day does it remain significantly under diagnosed? One of the reasons is probably the very distinctiveness of the "silver balls" or Pick bodies. It was not long before many, in fact the majority, of typical cases of Pick's disease (PiD) came to post-mortem examination not having typical Pick bodies. It turned out that there was a mismatch between what the clinicians diagnosed as Pick's disease and what the pathologists did. The Swiss neuropsychiatrists, Tissot and Constandinidis, suggested that PiD should be classified as having (A) Pick bodies, (B) only Pick cells (the ballooned neurons), or (C) none of the above, only the neuronal loss and gliosis. This ABC of Pick's disease was not followed by everyone however, and pathologists insisted on excluding the diagnosis of PiD when they did not see Pick bodies. Clinicians accepted their judgment as the "gold standard", in effect giving up the clinical diagnosis over time. This unfortunately resulted in the prevalent belief that Pick's disease is rare.

The other reason for the decreasing recognition of the disease was the ascendancy of Alzheimer's disease in the awareness of physicians and the media in the 1970's. The screening methods of epidemiology and the simplification of the diagnosis with the "mini-mental" examination often replaced the careful clinical assessment needed for the diagnosis of the multifaceted clinical pattern of Pick's disease. Textbooks on dementia fostered the idea that Pick's disease is mainly diagnosed on post-mortem and the myth that it is practically impossible to distinguish it from Alzheimer's disease. A large number were indeed lumped together with AD in scholarly articles or what is even worse, in studies of treatment.

Cases of Pick's disease without Pick bodies were renamed *frontal lobe dementia* by two influential European groups, who subscribed to the idea that the term Pick's disease should be reserved for histology with Pick bodies (Brun 1987; Neary, Snowden, et al. 1988). The Lund and Manchester groups deserve a great deal of credit for renewing interest in the disease and defining the behavioural abnormality in modern terms. However, restricting the diagnosis of PiD to those cases with Pick bodies resulted in the fractionation of the illness.

The emphasis on frontal lobes neglected the language presentation, which is described as a separate disease under the term Primary Progressive Aphasia, with its own extensive literature. Every new group describing a clinical or pathological variety was keen to introduce new terminology. This fractionation of the admittedly multifaceted entity and the emphasis on AD in dementia studies delayed the recognition that this is a relatively common and important disease, and it could be differentiated from AD while the patient is still alive.

The Lund and Manchester Groups demonstrated convincingly that the disease they eventually renamed frontotemporal dementia (FTD) is far from rare, but it occurs in an estimated 12-15% of the degenerative dementias, at a ratio of 1:6 to AD. Subsequent epidemiological studies in Cambridge, England, showed that FTD occurs as frequently as AD in the population under age 65 (Ratnavalli, et al. 2002). Nevertheless, this information is slow to get through to the majority of neurological, psychiatric and geriatric specialists, possibly because of the terminological confusion, but also because of the complexities of the diagnosis. True prevalence statistics are still lacking because of the difficulties in diagnosis and the limitations and expense of doing an accurate population survey. Population studies for dementia and AD did not even have categories for FTD/Pick's and autopsy studies were also biased because the brains collected were primarily from Alzheimer centres.

One of the significant changes in the last decade is the acceptance that the behavioural variety of the disease (FTD-bv) and primary progressive aphasia (PPA), as described by Mesulam (1982), have the same underlying biology and pathology and converge clinically. *Semantic dementia* was added as a separate entity because of its striking clinical presentation but it is now recognized that many patients will have the behavioural symptoms at the same time as, or shortly after, presentation. Almost all FTD/Pick's patients have some *aphasic* speech disturbance of the semantic or the agrammatic nonfluent type earlier or later on in their illness and mutism is a mid to end stage symptom in all. Recently the *movement disorders* called corticobasal degeneration (CBD) and Progressive Supranuclear Palsy (PSP) have also come to be considered part of the complex.

It was known from the 1930's that Pick's disease was at times associated with a movement disorder. It was called the Akelaitis variety, after the neurologist who wrote about it. In 1968 Rebeiz, a resident, Kolodny, a neurologist, and F.P. Richardson, the senior neuropathologist from Boston, described several patients with neuropathology and clinical symptoms that seemed unique. These patients had unilateral stiffness, in some ways similar to the more common Parkinson's disease, severe apraxia, "alien hand" and vertical gaze palsy. They also had aphasia and behavioural change, but the movement disorder dominated the description. The pathology was recognized by the authors to be similar to Pick's disease, especially the ballooned neurons or Pick cells. The description was practically ignored for twenty years, when it was rediscovered and renamed *corticobasal degeneration* because the pathology was both in the cortex and in the basal parts of the brain (the basal ganglia are concerned with coordinating movements among other functions). It also became evident that many patients with this pathology did not have the movement disorder, but had progressive aphasia, or FTD, or both, when they were seen in the clinic. Here was another puzzling disconnect between the name used for the disease and the underlying pathology. Cases of clinical Pick's disease turned up without Pick bodies, but had CBD pathology, and the reverse occurred too, i.e. clinical cases of CBD with Pick pathology. The best way one can make sense of this seemingly confusing state of affairs is to consider these varieties as part and parcel of the same disease. Nevertheless the resistance to do so continues for various reasons. A major one is inertia; cherished beliefs and concepts are difficult to change. People have a vested interest in a disease and terminology.

In 1964, another group, John Steele, J.C. Richardson, and Jerzy Olszewski, from Toronto, published the clinical and pathological characteristics of a syndrome they also considered unique. These patients also resembled Parkinson's disease because they developed rigidity, loss of posture, frequent falls, and immobility. They had a characteristic paralysis of the up-down gaze that the authors named "progressive supranuclear palsy" (PSP), because they believed the damage to the eye movement system was above the oculomotor nuclei. These patients also developed slurred speech, difficulty swallowing, and forced inappropriate crying and laughter. They would screw up their faces in a spastic grimace, their colour turning crimson, tears flowing uncontrollably. This is called *pseudobulbar palsy* and *pseudobulbar crying*. Pseudo here does not mean faking, but that damage is not in the nuclei of the "bulb" part of the brainstem that move the facial muscles, but somewhere higher in the nervous system that controls the evocation of these movements.

It became evident after a while that CBD patients not only develop vertical gaze palsy and the other clinical features of PSP, but the pathology and genetics also overlap. Sometimes even experienced clinicians cannot tell them apart and when they apply one clinical label, the pathology often proves it to be the other. Although pathologists tried to define and delineate the differences, there are too many similarities and transitory forms to dismiss the overlap. It is not immediately obvious why a couple of seemingly esoteric movement disorders should be considered on the same page as FTD/Pick's. However, there are also many cases, where FTD precedes the PSP symptoms (see the "Hero of Bolero") and CBD-PSP symptoms often appear later in the course of FTD and PPA (see Chapters 4, 17 and 19). Finally, as discussed below, genetically the two diseases are practically identical and the abnormally clumped tau in the nerve cells has the same biochemistry.

FTD is now the commonly used term for the overall syndrome, but it is also used for the behavioural presentation. In order to avoid this duplication, our group suggested *Pick complex* to preserve historical accuracy and to avoid the confusion surrounding the term "Pick's disease" (Kertesz, et al. 1994), and the Manchester group suggested *frontotemporal lobar degeneration* for the overall syndrome (Snowden, et al. 1996). There is still no universal agreement on what term to use, and Pick's disease is still favoured by lay support groups and many clinicians. Despite several "consensus" conferences, there is also some controversy concerning what should be included in the syndrome. Until recently some clinicians and pathologists were reluctant to accept a unifying biology that would qualify it for a disease entity. There is a great deal of vested interest in describing new disease categories and assigning new names to them. The increasing body of evidence, however, is in favour of the overlap of the various clinical components and the underlying pathological varieties (Kertesz, et al. 2003).

The discovery of abnormally phosphorylated tau protein in both Alzheimer's and Pick's disease clarified the nature of the silver staining inclusions, but their role in the causation of the disease remains disputed. In AD the role of amyloid (the beta protein variety) in senile plaques has gained predominance (the researchers who champion this are called the "Baptists") and the role of abnormal tau was considered causative by a minority of investigators (the "Taoists"). With the discovery of tau mutation as the major abnormality in FTD/Pick's, the balance of discussion moved toward the importance of abnormal tau metabolism. Most investigators try to integrate the various molecular abnormalities in the causation of illness, rather than consider them exclusive, although efforts to pinpoint a cause or trigger in degeneration require fractionation and identification of distinctive mechanisms.

Everybody has normal, soluble tau; it is one of the many structural proteins essential for the functioning of the nervous system. It stabilizes microtubular proteins and enables axonal transport, the shifting of chemicals along the nerve fibres, contributing to the integrity of neural transmission. Tau mutations alter microtubular binding and diseased tau is abnormally phosphorylated, aggregrating into the silver staining inclusions. Antibodies developed against it can identify abnormal tau, and it can also be separated by modern biochemical techniques such as gel electrophoresis, "Western blots", etc. Each variety has its chemical signature, but there is considerable overlap between them. Not all cases of FTD/Pick's, not even half, have abnormally aggregated and stained tau in their brain. The tau negative cases still may be "tauopathies" because Virginia Lee, Vicky Zhukareva and their collaborators (2001) suggested normal tau was missing or decreased in some cases

and this may be as damaging as having abnormal tau accumu-
lating in the cells.

The association of dementia with motor neuron disease (MND)
was described in scattered reports and in a larger series from
Japan (Mitsuyama 1984). Later some of the dementia was
specified as FLD (Neary, et al. 1990). Amyotrophic Lateral
Sclerosis (ALS) or Lou Gehrig's disease are other terms used
for MND. It also became evident that cases of dementia with
MND have ubiquitin positive, tau negative inclusions in the
cortex, which have been previously described in the motor neurons of the spinal cord in amyotrophic lateral sclerosis (ALS).
Ubiquitin, as the name suggests, is a ubiquitous by-product
of protein metabolism in the brain, and sometimes a marker
of disease. Cognitive and behavioural impairment has been
observed in ALS and some estimate it to be as high as 50%
(Lomen-Hoerth et al 2002). About 10% of cases of FTD and
PPA develop MND (Neary et al. 1990; Caselli, et al. 1993).

Recently, the ubiquitin positive tau negative inclusions
were found in many cases of FTD without clinical MND,
even in the familial form. In fact, a majority of cases, previously described as having "dementia lacking distinctive
histology" turn out to have these rather distinct inclusions,
also called FTD-MND type inclusions, or motor neuron disease inclusion dementia (MNDID) (Jackson, et al.
1996). It is probably the most common finding on autopsy in
cases of FTD/Pick complex (Hodges, et al. 2003; Munoz,
2003; Kertesz et al.2005.) In fact, 13 of the 24 cases in this
book came to autopsy and nine of them had the MND type
Ubiquitin positive, Tau negative inclusions. Very recently a
new protein labelled "TDP-43" was found in the tau negative

ubiquitin positive inclusions. A possible target for therapy, its role is yet to be discovered. The next chapter touches upon the genetic features of these protein abnormalities.

There is also preliminary evidence that the Tau positive pathology is more often associated with PPA and CBD/PSP syndromes, and the Tau negative variety with the behavioural presentation and semantic dementia. Should we look at these as at least two distinct diseases? Time and new research will probably tell. At this point the evidence for clinical and pathological overlap seems to be more convincing than a separation, at least to some of us.

Continuing research into the biology of these syndromes is needed to understand their relationship and how the various abnormalities cause the loss of function, cell degeneration, and brain atrophy. Although some of the biological changes have been uncovered, there are many gaps in our knowledge. Hopefully some of these will be bridged in time to provide treatment to alleviate symptoms, to stop the degeneration, or even reverse it. This may be a tall order, but it is our obligation to try to fill it.

Twenty-Two

Diagnosis and Genetic Counselling

MUCH OF THE DIAGNOSIS is based on a good history from a reliable caregiver. However, the diagnosis can be suspected when the patient walks into the clinic, as they are often garrulous, jocular, and inappropriately inquisitive, reading and touching everything. In fact, Bonita Stevenson, my administrative assistant, and Magdalena Carter, the social worker who runs the daycare program and our Pick Support Group, have become skilled diagnosticians through picking up on such behaviour. One of our patients was actually diagnosed in church by the spouse of another patient who observed his disinhibited, gregarious behaviour (he kissed strangers instead of shaking their hands after communion).

I often start the interview with the patient and the caregiver present together. This way I can observe the behaviour and interaction, see whether or not the patient has insight into their condition, and make sure the patient does not feel excluded. However, I usually have to separate them shortly after and continue with the caregiver alone to get an accurate history, unhindered by the presence of the patient who may be sensitive to what the caregiver says. During this time the patient can be examined with one of the screening instruments or have the language battery carried out if s/he is obviously aphasic. After the caregiver has had a chance to tell the complete story, the diagnosis is often evident for most varieties of FTD/Pick complex.

The physical and neurological examination will be helpful to uncover aphasia, apraxia, disinhibited behaviour, the movement (extrapyramidal) disorder, gaze palsy, unilateral hand rigidity, alien hand, slowing of the movements, evidence of motor neuron disease such as up-going toes, hyperreflexia and wasting and twitching of the muscles and tongue. It is also important to exclude or uncover other conditions. Meanwhile, the psychologist or social worker goes through the Frontal Behavioural Inventory with the caregiver. At the end we integrate the history with the examination and the brief cognitive tests that could be carried out.

The whole diagnostic process takes about an hour and a half and includes some counselling for the caregiver and the patient. Unfortunately, this is more time than most physicians can spend with a patient. We try to anticipate this by booking fewer patients, but at times the diagnosis is not evident from the referral note that may only say "cognitive problems." A second interview, after the neuroimaging is completed, is often necessary and most useful for finalizing the diagnosis and further counselling the family.

Neuroimaging, which can usually be carried within a month or two of the initial examination, consists of magnetic resonance imaging (MRI) and single photon emission tomography (SPECT) at our centre, but a computerized axial tomography (CAT) scan is often adequate for the initial diagnosis. Positron emission tomography (PET) scanning provides the metabolic profile of focal atrophy versus diffuse impairment. Although more accurate than SPECT, it is too expensive to use routinely. In questionable cases, however, the SPECT and PET may add weight to the differential diagnosis. The radiological report often misses focal atrophy and I make a habit of reviewing my own scans. However, to be fair to the radiologists, sometimes they are the ones who make the diagnosis by drawing attention to the frontotemporal atrophy. Some radiologists are quite knowledgeable and will diagnose Pick's disease on the basis of a CAT scan showing large frontal horns or focal shrinkage on the MRI. I find randomly reported SPECT scans by general imaging specialists less diagnostic, although in some centres patients are selected on the basis of SPECT scan for research. An electroencephalogram (EEG) is useful to exclude other diseases such as Creutzfeldt-Jakob (similar to "mad cow", but not caused by eating beef), epilepsy, or even Alzheimer's disease, which tend to have more abnormal EEG's than occur in FTD. Occasionally early neuroimaging does not show the focal atrophy and in those cases I rely on the clinical history and examination. Repeated neuroimaging, especially with MRI, provides a fairly accurate documentation of progressive focal atrophy and excludes underlying problems that could mimic FTD/Pick's disease, such as a slowly growing brain tumour. No diagnosis of FTD/Pick's disease should be considered accurate without at least a CAT scan or an MRI at the beginning of the illness and preferably repeated a couple of years later.

The diagnosis can be difficult in the very early cases when only partial loss of executive function creates inattention, inability to handle complex tasks or problem solving. Although the patient appears cognitively intact with good memory and normal behaviour, s/he is unable to carry on with their work. Early FTD cases with job failure may have occupational stress or "burn out" to blame as the cause of these symptoms, when in fact they are secondary to the loss of executive function. In these instances it is important to exclude depression, as this could be the cause of "job burn out" or inability to carry out household chores. A period of treatment with antidepressants is useful to exclude depression as a reversible cause of cognitive impairment (used to be called "pseudodementia").

Occasionally adult attention deficit disorder has similar symptoms. Personality and behavioural change after head injury can be quite similar, but it is clearly attributable to the injury, and therefore should not enter the diagnostic consideration. At times caregivers or primary physicians say the patient has loss of memory, which may be shorthand for inattention or disorganization. True early memory loss usually signifies Alzheimer's disease, but semantic dementia also interferes with memory testing.

Some of the early behavioural abnormalities could be attributed to pre-existing personality quirks. Somebody who had the obsessive compulsive personality trait before may not be faulted for obsessive shopping or preoccupation with elimination or with certain foods. Just about any behaviour described in this book can be observed in normal individuals in isolation, in a mild form or as a lifelong personality trait. How many of us are considered "pack rats" by our spouses? The selfish, inconsiderate, childish character of

George Constanza on "Seinfeld" is a comic example of the "normal" version of the "frontally challenged" personality. Nevertheless, in most instances the recent emergence and the excessive, bizarre nature of these behavioural abnormalities provide clear evidence for the disease for those who are aware of it. The emphasis should be on the change from previous personality or behaviour.

We constructed and standardized a Frontal Behavioural Inventory (FBI) to facilitate the diagnostic process and to measure the severity of the change. The caregiver is asked questions in a positive and negative way so as not to bias them in either direction (Kertesz et al. 1977). Although caregivers differ in their ability to be objective about their charges, most of the time we obtain a rather accurate picture from the scores. Occasionally they tend to protect the patient and underestimate the severity of the behaviour, but almost never ever exaggerate. The FBI explores 24 behaviours. The first 12 questions about apathy, aspontaneity, indifference, inflexibility, personal neglect, disorganization, inattention, loss of insight, decreased speech (aphasia), alien hand (apraxia), and semantic errors are "negative" in the sense of decreased function.

The positive symptoms are perseverations, obsessions, irritability, jocularity, poor judgment and impulsivity, hoarding, inappropriate remarks, restlessness, aggression, hyperorality and food fads, hypersexuality, utilization behaviour and incontinence. The caregiver scores these as none, mild, moderate, or severe representing a change from before the illness. Most patients who have FTD score 27 or above and most patients who do not, score below that. After the first publication of this test (Kertesz, et al. 1997) further standardization has been carried out, supporting its reliability and utility.

There are translations in French, German, Italian, Hungarian, Portuguese and Spanish.

Some of the verbal behaviours, disinhibition, apraxia, utilization behaviour and aphasia can be observed during the neurological examination. Other tests of frontal lobe functions have been constructed to elicit impairment of motor sequencing, preservation and a variety of executive functions: Frontal Assessment Battery (FAB) (Dubois, et al. 2000), or cognitive flexibility (Card-sorting or the "Stroop-test") or multitasking and attention (Trail-Making) or planning and working memory (The tower of Hanoi). Performance on these "frontal tests" can be surprisingly normal, however, in behaviourally disturbed or aphasic FTD patients.

Neuropsychological testing at early stages is useful to differentiate FTD from AD by documenting the relatively preserved memory and visuospatial function in FTD/Pick's while these are significantly impaired in AD. Language and "frontal lobe executive" tasks are more severely affected in FTD. Language testing is useful to document the severity and the loss of fluency in PPA that distinguishes it from the milder language impairment in AD in the middle stages. The so-called "executive function" of planning, problem-solving and multitasking may or may not be impaired. Furthermore, executive function tests are the least specific because executive function is also affected early in AD or, in fact, in any brain damaged patient.

In mid-stages it is more difficult to differentiate patients by using neuropsychological testing since FTD patients are restless and often uncooperative. A complete neuropsychological battery is time consuming, tiring, and difficult to standardize. If the wrong tests are selected, misdiagnosis is common, especially if someone unaware of the characteristic patterns does the testing and interpretation. Patients at later stages become untestable with the detailed and more sensitive measures and short screening tests are not specific to differentiate the various dementias by their overall scores. In these stages the differential diagnosis is heavily dependent on good history, observation, examination and neuroimaging.

Primary progressive aphasia (PPA) is more often referred to neurologists, while the behavioural variant tends to be referred to psychiatrists for diagnosis. The aphasic presentation is gradual and the exact mode of onset is very important to determine. Sudden or rapid onset of aphasia is almost always due to a stroke or some infectious disease but a slowly progressive aphasic syndrome is either related to FTD/Pick's disease or a slowly growing brain tumor and neuroimaging is absolutely essential to rule these out. Furthermore neuroimaging is useful to diagnose FTD/Pick's with focal atrophy. The other important differential diagnosis is Alzheimer's disease (AD) because it also may have a significant aphasic component. However, when Alzheimer patients become aphasic it is usually at a later stage of their illness and by that time they have considerable loss of memory. Patients who begin with word finding difficulty and develop progressive loss of language without the memory and visuospatial difficulties are more likely to have PPA. A skilled clinician can make the diagnosis relatively easily if the caregiver is reliable and observant, especially regarding the onset of changes, and if the examination is thorough. A formal language test such as the Western Aphasia Battery (WAB) (Kertesz 1982) helps to determine the extent and type of language disturbance, especially measuring the loss of fluency which is the most important feature in PPA. In contrast, impaired language in AD tends to remain fluent.

Patients with semantic aphasia form a special group because their language disturbance is unique and dramatic, consisting of the multimodality loss of meaning. Alzheimer patients rarely, if ever, lose the meaning of things so early. AD patients have word finding difficulties and later on they may have comprehension difficulty and semantic errors, but they do not ask for the meaning of words heard in conversation. The loss of comprehension and inability to recognize objects can be the presenting symptom in semantic aphasia and repeated questioning of the meaning of words is diagnostic. Subsequently, it is almost invariably associated with the behavioural abnormality and this also distinguishes it from AD. Sometimes the caregivers are struck by the bizarre questioning of the meaning of ordinary words (what is "steak") and sometimes they dismiss it as part of the jocularity and may or may not talk about it. We incorporated this into the FBI questionnaire to remind the caregivers.

The most common psychiatric differential diagnosis is between FTD/Pick's disease and depression or a bipolar manic-depressive illness. The apathy, aspontaneity, indifference, and inattention of Pick's disease, however, is quite different from the apathy, anhedonia (inability to enjoy), visible sadness, crying, thoughts of worthlessness and suicide, and the sleep disturbance that characterize true depression. FTD patients hardly ever cry or feel sad, they are indifferent to their disease and as a rule appear emotionally flat. Furthermore, they do not have the typical sleep disturbance of early awakening. We use depression inventories such as the Cornell Depression Scale (obtained from caregivers) or the Beck Depression Scale (directly from the patients) to exclude depression. In difficult (usually early) cases we often obtain a psychiatric consultation for a second opinion. It is important to treat patients for depression if there is any doubt. Nevertheless, borderline, mixed or questionable cases turn up, especially in a referral clinic. Such a diagnostic dilemma is described in Chapter 15 where an obsessive/compulsive disorder may be combined with manic-depressive psychosis to mimic FTD. Diagnostic issues are different in each stage of the illness. Usually within two or three years of the onset of the illness there is sufficient evidence to make an accurate diagnosis. However, in the end stages the symptoms of degenerative disease converge and it is more difficult to make the diagnosis later on when the patient is incapacitated in many domains of cognition and mobility.

GENETIC COUNSELLING

After the diagnosis is made, genetic counselling may become important because FTD/Pick's disease is more often dominantly inherited than AD. Even though many Alzheimer patients have another family member who has died with some type of dementia or "senility", the incidence of age-related memory loss and the combination of AD and vascular disease is so high that this kind of family occurrence does not mean a diagnosable genetic pattern. In contrast, FTD/Pick's disease has a relatively high number of families with a Mendelian dominance where the disease is passed on from generation to generation. Mendel was a German priest-scientist with considerable gardening skills, who crossed white and black flowering peas to establish the classical rules of dominant and recessive inheritance (you may call him the father of genetic engineering). Dominant means that if you have a parent with the illness, you have a 50%

chance of inheriting it. The flip of the coin applies to everyone individually; in other words, it does not matter how many siblings may or may not be affected, each child has a 50% chance of inheriting the illness.

This kind of pattern is often linked to certain chromosomes and genes and in the case of FTD/Pick's disease, a large family was linked to chromosome 17 by Wilhelmsen and his collaborators (Wilhelmsen, et al. 1994). To establish such a linkage with certainty, fairly large families with several generations of affected members are needed and blood is taken from both affected and unaffected members. Wilhelmsen knew that the tau gene is located on chromosome 17 (along with many others of course) and suspected it to be the culprit, but the discovery of tau mutations was left to others (Hutton et al, 1998). Soon tau mutations were found in about half of the chromosome 17 linked families. With a tau mutation the abnormality can be detected in the affected individual and the same abnormality could be looked for in their unaffected siblings or offspring to predict whether they are carriers of the mutation and whether or not they will develop the disease. Sequencing the tau gene to detect mutations, however, is not a routine procedure, and is carried out in only a few research laboratories.

Many family members ask me about the chances of them or their children getting the disease. I usually explain it in the following manner: Approximately 30-40% of FTD/Pick's disease is familial. Linkage to chromosome 17 can be found in fewer than half these families. Half of those with linkage may have a mutation in the tau gene. So far no mutation has been found in sporadic or single cases. Therefore, our current practice is to look for a mutation only in those families where more than one member is affected and the pattern is dominant (from generation to generation). Often people do not have information on relevant family members such as siblings, uncles, and cousins. A certain amount of telephoning, inquiring about details and discrete detective work is a worthwhile exercise for any family affected by FTD/Pick's disease. When a dominant pattern is documented, we, in collaboration with a genetic laboratory, will look for a mutation, but even then, the chances of finding one are variable, around 10%. Once we have found a mutation in an affected individual it is up to each family member to decide whether or not they want to have their blood examined. Not being a carrier of a mutated gene is a great relief, of course, and ensures that your offspring are safe. Knowing either way helps family planning. Most people would want to know, although there are some who have their reasons not to and genetic counselling in a confidential manner is helpful. I usually ask the relatives of my patients to do some homework and prepare a family tree for our next visit so that genetic counselling will be effective. Without such information, counselling is only tentative. I also suggest thinking of the implications of knowing or not knowing whether one is the carrier of a genetic abnormality that will almost certainly result in a disease later or may be passed on to offspring (a 50% chance).

The mutations are not necessarily specific for the clinical patterns. The most common mutation is the change of amino-acid proline to leucine on codon (coding region) 301 (P301L) of the tau protein, which may present with the behavioural, or the aphasic or the extrapyramidal motor disorder. Even in a single family the same mutation can cause different patterns. The pathology is not predicted by the mutation either. Certain mutations tend to produce either the CBD Pick variety, but certain mutations such as P301L produce all of the varieties. Tau negative cases are more common in FTD than in PPA or in the CBD/PSP syndrome.

The tau negative cases may be linked to other genetic loci such as chromosome 9 where the linkage in one family was associated with FTD-MND (same pathology as seen in the motor neurons of ALS (Lou Gehrig's disease). Very recently, just as this book goes to press, some of these families with tau negative pathology have been discovered to have mutations of progranulin (PGRN) which is also on chromosome 17, some distance from the tau gene. The search is on for the nature of the genetic interaction between these two protein mutations, causing similar if not identical illness and other linkages and mutations, to further clarify the genetic causation and diagnosis in families.

Twenty-Three

Notes for Caregivers

PROVIDING CONTINUING CARE for an FTD/Pick's patient must be the ultimate test of a person's character. The challenge of dealing with a spouse or a parent, who is becoming not only disinterested in work, family, friends, and normal conversation, but is actually changing to become a rude, childish, disinhibited, obsessive, and inflexible individual, is enough to break the spirit of many. It is an inspiring testimony to human compassion, to see how most of the carers overcome their initial bewilderment, fear, denial and anger and learn to cope. In this chapter I attempt to help the caregivers who were my inspiration and source of much of what is written here. Many self-help books and caregiver guides are available for Alzheimer's disease and much of that applies to this condition as well (the classic is called "The 36-Hour Day"). Support groups (see the end of the chapter) and supportive families help many carers. It is not my aim to provide

a detailed practical guide to meet all conceivable needs, but
to give a concise summary of useful advice for those common
problems that I found specific for the illness.

The illness comes insidiously and sometimes remains
unrecognized for years. Inability to get organized at work
or do complex tasks such as meal preparation or household
maintenance are early, but not specific, symptoms. The spouse
and relatives may wonder if it is just a "burnout", depression,
or stress at work, or at home. They use commonly known
terms and clichés inaccurately such as "memory loss" and
"depression". Loss of language and failure to recognize faces
and objects are often attributed to bad memory. These short-
cuts and interpretations of symptoms instead of a detailed
description of what the patient actually says or does may lead
to delayed or missed diagnosis.

Occasionally relatives choose to ignore the symptoms or
attempt to cover up the social consequences of the personality change by avoiding situations that lead to embarrassment,
and withdraw socially altogether. One of the spouses in my
practice, still very much in love with his youngish attractive
wife, stalwartly defended her behaviour even when their adult
daughters insisted something was very, very wrong. At times,
travel abroad or a move precipitates or highlights the difficulties dealing with change, upsetting routine or waiting. At other
times relatives, who have not seen the patient for a while, draw
attention to the personality change.

Tip #1: Don't blame "stress," or "cover up" (oh, it is just a phase) too
long, although finding excuses for your partner from kindness
is understandable.

The next step, after realizing the gradual change of personality is more than a temporary or transient symptom, is to obtain accurate diagnosis and help in management. Most patients with this illness totally lack insight and some stubbornly refuse to see a physician, let alone a psychiatrist. Sometimes it is helpful to find a more "organic" reason to go to the doctor and use the word "specialist" to avoid the suggestion of mental illness. Even when the patient is coaxed into going for a visit, they often say "there is nothing wrong with me." Sometimes they put up such resistance that the spouse makes the mistake of letting them go to the physician "for a checkup only", which leads to incomplete assessment, because the diagnosis of FTD depends on a reliable history from a spouse or someone close.

It is helpful for more than one family member to provide a perspective, a different angle on the development of the change, although too many people in the office may be difficult difficult to handle and time consuming for the physician or the psychologist. In our clinic we provide extra chairs for all comers if needed, but also try to interview the principal players separately. Not all clinics have this luxury of time, space and personnel. Until recently, the diagnosis of FTD has been made mostly by a few specialists and, believe it or not, by caregivers, by friends, and even through the Internet. Unfortunately, awareness of the diagnosis has not reached most general practitioners or other specialists yet. Hopefully this book and the efforts of FTD clinics and volunteer support associations will provide an impetus for better recognition.

Tip #2: Always accompany your charge to the physician's office and ask to speak to him/her alone if possible. This will be done in organized specialty clinics, but don't count on it everywhere.

It is useful to be prepared with a list of symptoms, behaviours, and personality change in order of development. Try to define the first symptoms, as they are the most diagnostic, even though most recent problems seem to be more pressing. Try to describe them in detail not just: "he can't do anything" or "meals are not what they used to be". Some physicians like to listen, some like to look at a brief concise list while you talk, and a few (I am one of them) welcome a longer, several pages of written tale of woes. Primary physicians may not have the time to read all that or to make sense of it, except to make a decision to refer. As you recount the symptoms glance at the doctor. If s/he seems to be short of time ask him if s/he would like a copy. S/He may be able to read it later.

The specialists most likely to be knowledgeable about the disease will be in the departments of neurology, psychiatry and geriatrics at a university or memory clinic or Alzheimer centre. Neurologists will likely see the language loss, (aphasic) presentation, but the behavioural-personality disorder will probably be referred to a psychiatrist. Memory is almost always preserved for episodes initially, although it may be lost for names and faces, and these people do not get lost like Alzheimer patients. Make sure you mention the sparing of these functions if that is the case, as they can be diagnostic at the beginning. In later stages even these functions become impaired or impossible to test, because of the behavioural change or the language loss.

Tip #3: Prepare a brief, one page list of symptoms, behaviours, and personality change and approximate dates in order of appearance. Try to get a referral to the top specialist in the area.

After obtaining the diagnosis, the questions begin to multiply. What caused it? Could it be something else? What is the course? Is there a treatment? Could it get better? The outcome? How long is the duration? Who else is affected? What can I do to help? How does it affect the family, myself? Is it hereditary? Where can I get help? What is the end like?

Sometimes these questions come out all at once, but mostly they occur to the caregiver later. The initial examination may not provide the diagnosis right away, let alone the answers to all of these questions. Some time is needed to collect the information from specialists, neuropsychologists, brain imaging scans, and laboratory tests. The family doctor may not feel ready to provide the answers and may leave it to the specialist to do all the integration and interpretation of complex data. General practitioners cannot be expected to be familiar with this disease yet, and this should not be held against them.

Often the diagnosis of manic-depressive illness is made, which is not necessarily a bad one, since the apathy, disinterest, and lack of spontaneity are similar to that is seen in depression and the disinhibition may resemble the manic phase. The modern serotoninergic (SSRI) type of antidepressants are, in fact, the treatment of choice so far, in FTD as well as in Obsessive Compulsive disorders (OCD). Most of the time the FTD/Pick's disease pattern is unmistakable for those familial with it, but borderline, difficult to diagnose cases stump even the best of experts.

TIP #4: Obtain information from several sources, including the Internet (see Tip 22). Continue to respect and maintain good relations with the family doctor no matter what the initial diagnosis.

Individual symptoms vary in order of appearance and
require different coping strategies. One of the first to
appear is apathy or lack of motivation. Disinterest in the
family, friends, social activities or previous hobbies can be a
striking change. Indifference, detachment, lack of motivation should be recognized as part of the disease and not
taken personally by the caregiver. Apathy or lack of interest is commonly mistaken for depression, or "burnout", but
it should be evident that the person is not sad or suicidal,
just disinterested. It is the least specific of the FTD/Pick
behaviours and is seen in Alzheimer's or vascular disease as
well. The apathy and indifference of FTD/Pick's are usually resistant to antidepressants, but it is worth trying them.
Caregivers coping strategies vary. Gentle reminders may
work at the beginning, bribery at midstages, and having
somebody else to do the chores eventually. Sometimes brib-
ing a reluctant patient with an ice cream cone does wonders to get them to the doctor or to do something. Angry
recrimination or nagging does not work at any stage. There
is a whole range of behaviours from laziness through apathy
to "abulia", which is the psychiatric term to indicate when
the patient's responsiveness and activity level is pathologi-
cally, unquestionably below the norm.

TIP #5: **Reminders to do things should be gentle. Rewards may be
more effective than confrontation. Get somebody else to do the
chores later. Try to involve family and friends to provide structure and stimulation.**

Impaired judgment, particularly concerning money and financial responsibilities, may be an early change, but has serious consequences. FTD patients are easy targets for T.V. ads, magazines, the internet, or mail order advertising, and some compulsively enter every giveaway contest or buy lottery tickets. It is amazing how easily FTD patients get on "sucker lists" as their poor judgment makes them easy prey to scams. Door-to-door solicitation for new windows or siding can result in substantial, unnecessary expenditure. Sometimes money is given away to charities by patients who can ill afford it. Telephone solicitation may be avoided by the use of answering machines with a short "fuse". Once the caregiver becomes aware of this, steps should be taken depending on individual situations, but a voluntary power of attorney to act on behalf of the patient should be sought early. It is difficult to declare a person, who is relatively intact cognitively, financially incompetent and officially certified competency examiners may not be aware of this early aspect of the illness. At this stage patients are often able to rationalize and convincingly excuse their spending and may resist interference. A valid Power of Attorney (POA) document transferring financial and health decisions to a spouse or a child can prevent much trouble later. A POA can be given to any relative or trusted friend in a simple form that is legally binding. To avoid battles between caregivers a little understanding earlier can prevent a lot of misunderstanding later. The different types of POAs vary between jurisdictions, but when obtained while the patient is in good health, they remain in force and are available when needed.

TIP #6: **Impaired judgment and financial irresponsibility can be costly. Obtain a power of attorney early if you can, speak to the bank manager, cancel unnecessary credit cards and contracts.**

Another form of impaired judgment, combined with impatience and impulsivity, commonly leads to driving errors. Cutting others off, hesitating, taking chances, misjudging distances and disregarding the needs of others appear earlier than errors of the mechanics in driving or the operation of a vehicle. Minor accidents are common, and sooner or later this may become a major issue with the behavioural variety of presentation. FTD patients rarely admit to any problems and may even pass driving tests. Males particularly may fight tooth and nail to hang on to their car, and even drive without a licence. One patient from my practice was killed on his motorcycle a month after he managed to convince another physician that he was healthy and fit to drive. Others can be persuaded to hand over their keys, and be "promoted" to be "copilots" or "navigators". Caregiver observations are critical to discontinue driving in time to prevent accidents. Progressive aphasics on the other hand often continue to drive well into their illness, as they are less likely to have impulsivity and impaired judgment. Prohibiting such a person from driving can unnecessarily curtail their personal freedom and causes grief and anger.

Tip #7: **Driving discontinuation is a significant step and the caregiver has an important role to make sure it is done as soon as it is necessary, but not before.**

Food fads and gluttony are frequent and typical symptoms. Simple restriction of availability may work, but patients often buy, pilfer, hoard, and hide their favourite sweets or snacks. Sometimes the extent of insistance on eating certain types of food becomes obsessive, to the exclusion of ordinary meals.

Addiction to bananas is particularly common, featured in several of the chapters. Bananas are harmless and have high nutritional value. Banana craving may have a physiological basis, since bananas contain abundant tryptophane, a precursor of serotonin. Serotonin deficiency is postulated to play a role in obsessive-compulsive and restless behaviour. Sweet craving could be a sign of diabetes, especially when accompanied by excessive drinking of water and frequent washroom visits; blood sugar should be checked. Gluttony can reach an alarming extent and cause weight gain, but it can be controlled by smaller servings. Occasionally compulsive drinking is a feature, not to be mistaken for alcoholism.

Tip #8: Food fads are harmless, but try to limit sweets without entering into an argument. Ask your doctor about if diabetes could possibly be causing this.

Stereotypic, recurrent routines are common and mostly benign, but insistence on doing the same thing, at the same time, day in and day out, can be wearing. Most caregivers find it easier to give in to tolerate the behaviour, as long as there is no interference with neighbours or strangers, etc. The frequent telephone habit is particularly difficult to take and may necessitate restriction of phone access. Obsessions with shopping, money, elimination, health, and body parts all require different strategies of coping and some may consume energy and time. Caregivers may have to limit access to shops and sales, take away credit cards, and control bank accounts. One of the caregivers in our support group successfully persuaded her husband to hand over his credit cards one by one by point-

ing out the duplication of the two of them having the same
card, and how too many cards lead to confusion. Getting off
mail order lists may not be as easy. Some patients stubbornly
resist any change in their routines and caregivers may have to
give in, or use clever, sometimes devious distraction strategies,
bargaining and bribery to avoid anger and confrontation.

TIP #9: Tolerate most obsessive routines if they are harmless.
Try to distract the person if their behaviour is disruptive.
With any luck, you can capitalize on creative obsessions,
such as crafts, jigsaw puzzles and painting to keep them
safely occupied for a while.

Roaming the neighbourhood, or the malls, often ventur-
ing long distances is disturbing and it overlaps with obsessive-compulsive behaviours. The behaviour is purposeful and
stereotypic, not like the agitated, confused wandering of AD
patients. FTD patients, in contrast to AD, do not get lost
and as a rule it is safe to let them roam, up to a certain extent.
Going for long walks is even healthy as long as they stay on
familiar streets, or on rural roads. It is recommended to check
out their route and have a general idea of their whereabouts.
Those who live alone or whose roaming is combined with
poor judgment or inattention, may get into trouble if they use
the shoulder or medians of busy highways or railroad tracks.
Some are restless and want to go to the mall daily or drive
long distances to their favourite restaurant. One caregiver I
know has given in and drives up to 150 km. a day with her
husband. Another patient ended up in California 3,000 miles
away without letting his spouse know. Some caregivers get

into a battle to discontinue the driver's licence or to confiscate keys to stop the roaming and this could precipitate a crisis.

> TIP #10: **Let them roam as long as they are safe. Try to distract them or go with them if you can. Sometimes it helps to say, "You don't need to drive there dear…" and change the topic or find something else for them to do.**

FTD/Pick patients often cannot sit still and will jump up from the dinner table or from a group conversation, due to short attention span. This may alternate with apathy or lack of spontaneity in the earlier stages of the illness. Restless pacing at home or clapping of hands, banging on walls and tables, usually comes at later stages, and is best handled by a verbal or action related distraction. Instead of saying, "Stop that, it drives me crazy", ask them to do something or tell you something (if they are still verbal). Restless behaviour can be so disruptive, that medication may be needed to cope with it. At times Selective Serotonin Reuptake Inhibitors (SSRI type of medications), or neuroleptics (tranquilizers) are useful for both restlessness and roaming. "Trazodone" has sedative and serotoninergic properties and may be particularly useful for some of these behaviours.

> TIP #11: **Minor degrees of restlessness or pacing do not need to be treated. However, if restlessness becomes disruptive or dangerous, medication may be helpful. Ask your doctor about it.**

Utilization behaviour, or picking up objects, utensils, etc. and using or fiddling with them, or just touching everything, is similar to restlessness. Some of this is tolerable such as rear-

ranging shelves or towels, but some of it is socially unacceptable– pilfering, touching other people's utensils or using every
container, even boots, boxes and glasses to urinate in instead
of the washroom. One spouse tried to cope by removing all
empty boxes, containers, etc., but eventually medication was
needed to stop this. Touching strangers, fiddling with the
clothes of others, patting children may create situations that
require quick pulling away or explanation if necessary. Another
somewhat similar behaviour is hyperorality, or not only touching, but tasting and putting everything in their mouth. This is
often a later stage phenomenon, and can be difficult to control
by verbal dissuasion.

**TIP #12: Most utilization behaviour is harmless. Warn your friends
before visits, speak to store clerks if necessary.**

Hoarding, pilfering, or shoplifting can be part of compulsive behaviour, but along with gluttony, utilization behaviour
or childish, selfish greed, all are considered to be under the
umbrella of disinhibition or failed social control. Caregivers to
keep an eye on their charge while shopping, and by explaining
to the store clerks what may happen before they are caught.
Some cope by avoiding stores, but if patients are on their own,
the caregiver should be prepared for this "asocial behaviour".
It is not "kleptomania", which is a compulsion occurring in
younger people, and it is not done for need unless it is for sweets
or snacks. Identification of the patient as a Pick sufferer and a
short note, explaining that he may touch or take things compulsively (make sure you use this explanatory adjective) because
of his illness, may help to prevent a nasty confrontation or

prosecution. Since few people know about Pick's disease, an Alzheimer bracelet may be a reasonable, if inaccurate substitute, and it is easily available.

TIP #13: **Beware of shopping malls. If you cannot watch him/her or forewarn people, a note with or without a "medic-alert" bracelet with your phone number and "Pick's disease" (or "Alzheimer's disease", since it is better known) may save a lot of trouble.**

Childish jocularity, singing, or dancing in public, smart-alecky remarks, cutting lines, rudeness, risqué or sexually charged behaviour are various degrees of disinhibition or failed social control and cannot be easily treated or prevented. Walking up to strangers, especially children, can be problematic and needs to be discouraged gently, but emphatically, or controlled by distraction. Hypersexuality is rarely a physical problem, but in the case of younger patients the actual increase in sexual demands may be difficult for some spouses to adjust to. In most cases it is mostly dirty jokes or remarks, occasionally touching or lifting clothes in public. This is rarely threatening, because this behaviour from a middle-aged or older person is so bizarre. Targets do not usually feel victimized, but may be surprised or walk away or go along with the joke. However, there may be less tolerance of any sexual aberration nowadays. Equally, if not more disturbing, is the loss of true intimacy, sexual, or spiritual.

TIP #14: **Prepare to be embarrassed by disinhibited behaviour, but remember s/he is a sick person. Angry, punishing words create similarly angry reaction and guilt on your part, and often will not modify this behaviour. Tolerate most of it if you can (it helps to have a thick skin), drag her/him away**

with a few words of explanation to the victim if you are
there. Ask for SSRI or tranquillizing medication from
your doctor.

Stubborn rigidity, resistance to change and contrariness may
occur and are best handled by distraction and avoiding confrontation. Easier said than done, but most caregivers manage
to do an excellent job and avoid arguments. It can be a real
challenge to cope with a stubborn, irritable, contrary FTD or
for that matter Alzheimer (for whom this is common at mid–to
end-stage) patient whose nastiness may make you forget s/he
was your spouse or a parent in better times. It is as if you were
forced to live with a stranger who behaves like s/he was from
another planet, whose habits are not like yours, who is not
the person you knew. This can be depressing to the caregiver,
resulting in "burnout," and feelings of abandonment and anger.
Spouses of FTD/Pick patients are often treated for clinical
depression, and one I heard about committed suicide. Others
separate or divorce the patient, fortunately an infrequent happening in my practice. Caregivers must be aware of their own
stress level, and their mental, physical and social needs. Respite
care for a few weeks, if it can be arranged, or other forms of
relieving caregiver burden must be sought regularly.

Tip #15: When the going gets rough and you feel you are at the end of
your rope, try sitting down with a cup of tea, or go to his/her
favourite doughnut shop and remember the good times spent
with him/her.

Coping with anger and guilt are probably the most difficult challenges a caregiver will face, even beyond the increasing physical and time demands. Being angry with a socially inappropriate individual who is childish, rude, or selfish is a natural reaction. Anger is counterproductive however, and its expression will not modify FTD behaviour. Remind yourself several times a day: one does not yell or show anger to a sick person! The difficult skill a good caregiver develops is not to express anger, but at the same time understand the reasons for it and not feel guilty about these feelings. Guilt, helplessness and associated depression in caregivers are common and can be severe, requiring professional help. A caregiver may turn to a family doctor, social worker, clergy, local Alzheimer groups, which may be able to help or refer for expert help to cope with the "triple whammy" of anger, guilt and depression. FTD/Pick's is often said to impact caregivers more than the patient (who more often than not remains blissfully unaware). Some caregivers need professional counselling; others have the support of adult children, siblings or friends. It has been said wisely: every caregiver needs a carer. Support groups can go a long way in providing this role.

Tip #16: Bite your lip! Control your anger by reminding yourself that s/he is sick and one does not yell at a sick person. Turn away while you collect yourself and think of something neutral to say or say nothing and distract the individual from the unacceptable behaviour. If you can't control your anger and guilt, ask for help.

Many of the FTD behaviours are strange; some are even funny and with a sense of humour are easier to take. Just like you smile at a child who comes out with an abrupt, candid remark, or insists on having his favourite snack or activity, you can try to see the humour in the bizarre twists of behaviour in this new person you have to live with. Roll your eyes and laugh, preferably when s/he cannot see you. Go to the video store to rent "As Good As It Gets" starring Jack Nicholson to see how many of the portrayed obsessive-compulsive and asocial behaviours are familiar. Talk to other caregivers of FTD patients; humour is infectious. I have heard it said: "Nothing like a shared laugh to brighten your day".

TIP #17: **Keep your wits about you. Find your sense of humour if you can when something funny happens, even though at first you may feel exasperated. Share your experience with others and you may get comforting feedback.**

Communication may be impaired in complex and initially subtle ways such as rambling, interrupting others and wanting to talk about only certain favourite topics. This impairment of the communicative rules of language is beyond phonology/articulation, grammar/fluency, and meaning/semantics. It has to do with give and take in conversation, staying on topic, responding to the point, coherence, and relevance, collectively called the "pragmatic" features of language. This kind of subtle but pervasive difficulty in communicating with an FTD patient can be a striking and early phenomenon, not quite as disturbing as others, but contributing to the impression of profound personality change; after all, communication is an important component, if not the essence of personality. Don't take it personally if s/he interrupts or does not understand you or does not follow conversation. Warn others about the communication problem, the lack of normal give and take, perseverating with certain topics and bizarre responses.

TIP #18: Interrupting conversations, not listening, perseverating with certain topics may be the first signs of the illness and may cause the loss of high level jobs. Be prepared for social isolation as a result.

Language may be impaired early or may even be the first thing to go. This can take various forms. Initially, patients seem to talk less and not join in conversation. There are others who develop stuttering or stumbling of speech but whose comprehension is preserved, and some have better writing. (These cases may be called primary progressive aphemia or verbal apraxia). Patients may become mute early while they are still quite capable of doing chores, taking care of others, or even continuing to work at their jobs. Those with decreased speech output and grammar and relatively preserved comprehension and cognition are described as having primary progressive aphasia (PPA). Some will not have any behavioural abnormality until later in the course of their illness, but the motor clumsiness (apraxia) and the development of a useless rigid hand (corticobasal degeneration syndrome) are commonly associated. A great deal of patience may be required to listen to a PPA patient search for a word. Sometimes they dislike someone else coming up with the word, but others welcome a helper who supplies the word they are struggling for. A patient listener who occasionally helps with cueing is probably the best for most. Phrasing a question so that a simple "yes" or "no" answer is required can help.

Try not to show frustration when the answer is not forthcoming. If you run out of time reassure them you will find out later. Try not to say "it does not matter", because it probably matters to them. At later stages their voice may be reduced to a whisper or they may echo what is being said. Sometimes verbal cueing such as saying: "The answer is"... helps. "Thumbs up" or "thumbs down" are useful signs to communicate, i.e. "Give me a thumbs up if you need the toilet." Holding an imaginary microphone works for others to coax some residual speech out of the aphasic, or almost mute individual. Be careful what you say in front of them. They usually understand more than they can vocalize.

TIP #19: Patients with PPA are often frustrated and depressed because of their decreasing ability to express themselves, but count your blessings, because they are much easier to live with for awhile, than other varieties of FTD/Pick patients. Simplify your questions so they require single word answers. Provide them a notepad and a pen, or a communication board with pictures to point to. Guessing what they want helps. Their driving need not be restricted until other symptoms develop.

Other forms of communication difficulty include the loss of meaning of things such as when a patient begins asking, "What is steak?" or a "parade?" or a "wall?" When comprehension is impaired and the patient does not know the meaning of items that come up in a conversation, the diagnosis of semantic aphasia (dementia) may be made (semantics is the processing of meaning). Persistent questioning of the meaning of words is characteristic. Some patients (often after someone advises them to) begin to label objects in the room on yellow "stickies" or make word lists compulsively. This is not overly helpful. Gestural explanations or carrying out an action with a pantomime may be more effective. Not only do word finding difficulty and wrong words appear but the loss of comprehension makes communication eventually even more difficult than in PPA. In a way semantic dementia or aphasia is the opposite of PPA: these patients speak much more than they comprehend. Later they may not even recognize objects or people visually, therefore the problem is not only verbal. Compounding this difficulty is the frequent association with the behavioural abnormalities, roaming and food fads, which can come before or after semantic dementia. Later echolalia or repeating everything said, or perseveration with a favourite word such as "advantage" or "Texas" occurs.

> TIP #20: Semantic aphasia or dementia impairs comprehension and communication needs to be supplemented with gestures and nonverbal actions. Be prepared that later on, they may not recognize objects or people when they see them, although this actually may be an early symptom. Bizarre as it may seem, they are not putting it on! Use simple direct questions, avoid analogies or metaphors. Get their attention by a gentle touch and eye contact.

Movement disorder may come early in the illness and may take several forms. It often robs the person of his mobility. This may come as a blessing in disguise for the caregiver of a roaming, restless, hyperactive patient with compulsive routines. They will not be able to go to the mall, to hoard, to accost strangers, and commit the annoying social gaffes they used to. However, a new set of problems will have to be dealt with. They may need a walker if they have the rigidity and frequent falls of progressive supranuclear palsy (PSP). The bizarre nature of the "alien hand," interfering with movements or the severe inability to use ordinary objects, often baffles caregivers until a proper explanation is provided. The relationship to FTD/Pick's may not be recognized, and another diagnosis such as Corticobasal Degeneration (CBD) is given to confuse the caregiver even further. Unfortunately, the rigidity and the immobility do not respond to treatment with levodopa or other medications for Parkinson's disease in this CBD/PSP variety of Pick's, which may resemble Parkinsonism.

TIP #21: The commonly developing CBD/PSP varieties of Parkinsonism in FTD/Pick's disease create mobility problems that are often helped by a wheeled walker. Some modifications to the house (ramps, bathroom railings) may be needed. Later on a wheelchair may be necessary.

Progressive inability to use household appliances, telephone, television, VCR, and eventually utensils to eat food is associated with all varieties of FTD presentation, but particularly with the corticobasal/aphasic syndrome and it is sometimes termed progressive apraxia. At times, however, it is related to the poor recognition of the object due to semantic dementia.

TIP #22: Simple, but distinct labeling of appliances, coloured dots on a button to push and nonverbal gestural instructions help at times.

Neglect of personal hygiene may require a few reminders first, but later on it may become a source of frustration. Battling over showers or shaving or clean clothes may give way to the need for complete supervision of all needs. It can be most disturbing that some of these relatively younger people become incontinent early in their illness. They seem to lose the frontal lobe function of regulating urination and defecation. At first, regular reminders to go to the bathroom every two hours may prevent some of the problems. Some patients with apraxia have trouble cleaning themselves and those with semantic dementia may not recognize what feces is or what toilet paper is for, and cleaning them becomes part of caregiving, the ultimate challenge for some. Modern adult diapers are easy to use and solve some of the problems. Community Care Access Services (in Ontario) will help with home care. Voluntary organizations, such as the Alzheimer Society, churches, or Shriners, provide information about local resources and will loan wheelchairs, etc. Volunteers will stay with patients and many places offer respite care, in an effort to preserve the carer's sanity. In the United States most information about home care, institutional care, etc., comes through local area Agencies of Aging.

TIP #23: Take advantage of home care help and local Alzheimer societies or Agencies on Aging in the United States. Don't hesitate to ask and organize relatives and friends to spell you off for a few hours a day. They may save more than one soul!

Eventually the care of FTD/Pick patients becomes very difficult at home. This happens at variable times and for various reasons. Incontinence often tips the balance towards a nursing home. When around the clock, constant nursing care is required, or when a person becomes estranged and uncomprehending, nursing home care should be considered. At times the antisocial or dangerous behaviour precipitates psychiatric admission. Occasionally caregivers manage through to the end with the help of an extended family or community care nursing, supplemented by private nursing coverage, but even

the dedicated, healthy spouse who is willing to devote a lot
of physical and mental effort can reach a breaking point. At
times difficulty swallowing and choking shortens the course
of the illness. At some stage homecare becomes overwhelming, usually when incontinence, immobility, mutism, and
incomprehension set in. More often caregivers reach a decision
before those endpoints are reached. Although some caregivers
feel guilty about the relief they feel when the move occurs, the
patient often does not care and may be unaware of the change.
Many settle quite quickly in to their new environment; some
even find the company and the distractions to their liking.
Choosing a nursing home can be difficult, as there are many
factors to be considered, such as its proximity to family, the
quality of care and the facility itself. Physical care is only one
aspect of a nursing home. Continuing family involvement is
equally important.

TIP #24: **Consider a nursing home when you feel adequate care
can better be provided by professional caregivers. It
may take six months or more to find suitable accom-
modation, so look around well before the situation becomes impossible to manage.**

A great deal of comfort can be found in talking to other
caregivers who have gone through the same experience.
Caregivers realize that they are not alone, that their experience is not unique. They learn what help is available and pick
up tips to help with the burden of care. To take care of Pick
or Alzheimer patients has been described as "the Marathon
of Care". The "loneliness" of such a long distance run can be

eased considerably by support groups of kindred people with whom to share the experience and emotional burden.

Caregiver support groups specific for FTD/Pick's are now being formed at various major centres. Look for these at websites such as in England (www.pdsg.org.uk), and in the United States, the Association for Frontotemporal Dementias (www. FTD-Picks.org). The AFTD and the British organization are a good resource for brochures, newsletters, research updates, support group listings, conference information and advocacy. Many Alzheimer websites have a brief section on Pick's disease, some quite out of date and inaccurate. www.nih.pubmed and libraries will have technical information. University centres usually have somebody knowledgeable about FTD/Pick's disease in the departments of neurology, psychiatry, or geriatrics, or inquiry at the above websites can direct a caregiver to the right source.

When the end comes, many caregivers find a brain donation to one of the research centers to be the best gift to other Pick sufferers who are still alive.

TIP #25: Join a support group locally. When the end comes, consider brain donation to a research group, which may improve the plight of future Pick sufferers. An autopsy is important to confirm the diagnosis, and it helps to answer questions about heredity. It also contributes to essential knowledge and scientific information about the disease.

Twenty-Four

What Are We Doing about FTD/Pick's? Treatment Options and Research Directions

RECENT DISCOVERIES OF THE NEUROTRANSMITTER deficiencies in Alzheimer's disease led to the development of medications to improve the symptoms of Alzheimer's disease. These drugs, called cholinesterase inhibitors, improve cognition and behavioural symptoms to a modest degree, occasionally more dramatically, for a limited period of time. Whether they modify the course or the outcome of the disease, we are as yet unable to tell; there are studies to suggest that they may, but long-term studies are needed to be certain. Three of these drugs, Donepezil, Rivastigmine, and Galantamine have been approved for mild to moderate AD in most countries. Other drugs such as Memantine are approved for moderate to severe AD and several others are being researched.

There is also evidence for impairment of several neurotransmitter systems in FTD/Pick's disease. Cholinergic, Serotonin and Noradrenaline binding are decreased in PiD in affected cortical regions. The decreased Serotonin binding could be related to obsessive-compulsive symptoms, over-eating, food preferences for bananas, sweet cravings, and weight gain observed in some patients with PiD/FTD/Pick complex. Other behavioural impairments such as apathy and irritability, and the relative preservation of memory are also compatible with serotoninergic dysfunction. Selective sero-tonin reuptake inhibitors (SSRIs) have been tried in an open label application in FTD patients, improving some of the obsessive symptoms (Swartz, Miller, et al. 1997). Trazodone has been found to be efficacious in a placebo cross over design to improve behaviour in FTD (Lebert & Pasquier 1999). Cholinesterase inhibitors have not been tried sys-tematically and anecdotal reports of worsening or improve-ment are not reliable. Small doses of atypical antipsychotics (Neuroleptics) are effective in coping with the restlessness, roaming, and asocial behaviour. Much of the current treat-ment is only symptomatic; so far no drugs have shown to modify the course or duration of the disease.

We have carried out several drug trials in our institu-tion, including one with Lithium that has been shown to dephosphorylate tau in laboratories. Unfortunately, sever-al of the patients put on Lithium had side effects with no improvement. Therefore, we abandoned this open label trial. Similarly, a pilot study with Cerebrolysin infusion (containing nerve growth factor-like substance) failed to show significant improvement in PPA patients. We have undertaken a formal trial of Galantamine (Reminyl) with a cohort of FTD and PPA patients. Reminyl is a cholinesterase inhibitor, already approved for Alzheimer's disease, with some additional effects such as serotonin and dopamine release through presynaptic nicotinic receptor modulation. Unpublished results suggest some efficacy in the aphasic variety of FTD. Treated patients did not decline as much as those on placebo. Other drugs on trial for Alzheimer's Disease that could be applicable to other degenerative diseases such as FTD/Pick's are Glutamate channel inhibitors, nerve growth factors, stimulants, antioxidants, tau phosphokinases etc., but there is no evidence for their efficacy as yet. They have been tried in a few patients only and await formal, placebo controlled clinical research, with meaningful endpoints.

Future directions of research are likely to follow multiple paths that are clinical, neuropathological, biochemical and genetic. Clinically improved definition of the disease and increased diagnostic accuracy with improved neuroimaging and possibly biological markers in the blood or the cerebrospinal fluid (CSF) will help basic science to target research and to find populations for treatment trials. The sooner it is recognized that this disease is not rare, the better are the chances of finding the cause and the treatment. The estimated prevalence ranges from 6-25% of dementias, which needs to be clarified with careful population studies, and series of postmortem examinations that collect a representative sample of pathology. Even brain banks, affiliated with Alzheimer centres, have a negative bias because they examine mostly Alzheimer brains. High estimates from centers interested in the disease may represent a positive bias, but these are probably closer to reality than the current level of underestimation due to general under-diagnosis. American, British, Canadian, European, and Japanese centres are beginning to collect large cohorts of patients with FTD/ Pick's and are enabling a better recognition of the disease.

The active collaboration of neurologists, psychiatrists, geri-
atricians, neuropathologists, and molecular biologists yields
the best research and hope for the future. True epidemiological studies cannot be carried out until recognition of the
disease becomes standardized and more reliable.

Further advances can be expected in the biology of tau,
ubiquitin and synuclein, proteins that produce different
clinical and pathological manifestations that range from
Alzheimer's disease to Parkinson's. FTD/Pick's disease has
distinct features and seems to have a specific relationship to
alterations in tau. One of the more important directions of
research is aimed at the tau negative cases, which constitute
about half, if not more, of FTD/Pick's disease. Currently
these are thought to be due to a possible deficiency of normal tau, but still producing a very similar illness to the tau
positive cases, where abnormally phosphorylated tau is precipitated. Therefore, both the tau negative and tau positive
cases may represent the same spectrum of pathology. This
needs to be confirmed and clarified further. Similarly, the
genetic pattern underlying both the tau positive and the
tau negative pathology and its relationship to the clinical
syndromes awaits further exploration and clarification. The
dominantly inherited tau negative families are related to
the recently discovered mutations in the progranulin gene
(Baker et al. 2006).

One should expect formal treatment trials in the future
even though FTD/Pick's patients are difficult to standardize
and examine. Various tests adapted from other neuropsychological purposes are being used. Specific tests of behaviour
such as the Frontal Behavioural Inventory (FBI) and of
language such as the Western Aphasia Battery (WAB) are

useful to quantitate some of the deficits in order to determine the efficacy of drugs. Similarly, neurological scales
for rating the Parkinsonian symptoms and global scales of
change are needed to detect improvement. Tests of frontal
"executive function" are applicable to a small segment of
patients diagnosed early, and may not be sensitive enough
in presymptomatic at-risk individuals, nor specific enough
to be diagnostic. As the disease worsens, they are less useful
to detect change, because they quickly reach a "floor effect"
and significantly affected patients cannot perform them any
more. The search is on for sensitive, specific and objective
markers of the disease, but so far nothing replaces a careful
history from a reliable caregiver, taken by an experienced
clinician, supported by neuroimaging.

To date, we are lacking a specific target drug that promises
disease modification instead of just symptomatic treatment.
SSRI's, cholinesterase inhibitors, and other psychotropic
drugs need to be tested formally with FTD/Pick patients.
On informal trials they have not shown dramatic results,
only symptom relief. Other drugs that modify tau metabolism, nerve growth factors, antioxidants, etc. are waiting
to be tried. The opportunity and the need for research are
great and so is the hope that in the not too distant future
more effective treatments or even disease modification can
be achieved. These research directions have been sum-
marized at the proceedings of a recent conference held in
London, Ontario (Canada) as a supplement to the Annals
of Neurology published in June 2003 (Kertesz et al. 2003).
Interested research groups are planning further yearly or
biannual conferences on this intriguing and often under-
recognized disease.

The last few decades or so have seen great strides in the study of the disease and its underlying pathology. The current advances in basic molecular biology are nothing if not spectacular. The mapping of the human genome was completed in 2003, and of the 23,000 genes 16,000 are in the brain and 6,000 are estimated to be brain specific. It is hoped that the current decades of discovery will soon be translated into decades of treatment, benefiting the significant number of those affected. Gene therapy and stem cell research are still in their infancy, but hold great promise, despite the controversy they have generated. If knowledge grows as explosively as in the past (doubling every 10-15 years according to some estimates), we may see the coming of therapies we have not even imagined.

GLOSSARY

In order of approximate frequency of use:
1. **Frontotemporal dementia(FTD)**
   Used for both the:
   1. Behavioral variant, in this case FTD-bv would be preferable.
   2. The overall disease.
2. **Frontotemporal Degeneration (FTD)**
   1. Used for all pathological variants.
   2. The abbreviation is the same as clinical FTD.
3. **Frontotemporal Lobar Degeneration (FTLD)**
   Lobar was added for the overall pathological designation to reserve FTD for the behavioural presentation.
4. **Pick's Disease (PiD)**
   1. The overall clinical syndrome, used less now, but preferred by many for simplicity and historical accuracy.
   2. Histologically defined entity, diagnosable only on autopsy, with silver and tau positive, round or oval inclusions in the cortex.
5. **Pick Complex (FTD/Pick)**
   Includes all the clinical syndromes and underlying pathological variants. FTD/Pick is also used throughout this book, combining 1 and 5 as a composite abbreviation.
6. **Primary progressive aphasia (PPA)**
   Slowly progressive aphasia before anything else develops. Alternate term: Progressive Nonfluent Aphasia (PNFA).
7. **Semantic dementia (SD)**
   A multimodality loss of meaning, difficulty with both comprehension and naming, especially nouns. Semantic aphasia is a suggested alternative.
8. **Corticobasal Degeneration Syndrome (CBDS)**
   Unilateral rigidity, immobility, apraxia, and the "alien hand", but many of these patients develop features of FTD and PPA. It overlaps with PSP (10).
9. **Corticobasal Degeneration (CBD)**
   1. Basal ganglionic and cortical silver and tau positive neuronal inclusions, glial plaques and ballooned neurons or "Pick cells" are characteristic.
   2. Also used as the clinical syndrome (like in 8).

10. **Progressive Supranuclear Palsy (PSP)**
    Defined by vertical gaze palsy, slowness, falling and dysarthria.
    The symptoms, pathology, tau biochemistry, and genetics overlap
    with CBDs(8) and CBD(9). Probably part of Pick Complex.
    Some prefer to keep it separate.

11. **FTD with Motor Neuron Disease (FTD/MND)**
    This was initially described as a clinical entity. Alternative term:
    ALS-Dementia.

12. **FTD-Motor Neurone Disease Inclusion type (FTD-MND)**
    Many cases of FTD with ubiquitin positive tau negative inclu-
    sions, typical of MND, but most have no clinical MND. Also
    called Motor Neuron Disease Inclusion Dementia (MNDID).
    Probably the most common pathological variety of the Pick
    complex.

13. **FTLD-U**
    Frontotemporal Lobar Degeneration with Ubiquitin histology.
    Same as 12.

14. **FTDP-17**
    Frontotemporal dementia and Parkinsonism linked to chromo-
    some 17. Less than half of these families have tau mutations.
    The first published family also had amyotrophy (wasting, like
    in ALS). Other families have FTD, PPA, CBD, PSP, ALS in
    various combinations.

15. **Dementia Lacking Distinctive Histology (DLDH)**
    Pathology without Pick bodies or typical CBD features. Most of
    these turn out to have MND type inclusions when looked for.

16. **Argyrophillic Grain Disease, ALS-Parkinsonism-Dementia
    complex, ("Lytico-Bodig") of Guam, Mesial Temporal Sclerosis,
    Neuronal Intermediate Neurofilament Disease (NIFID),
    Progressive Subcortical Gliosis, Tangle only Dementia**
    These pathological entities of uncertain position are considered to
    be part of the Pick complex by some, one time or another. Their
    clinical correlates need to be clarified.

References

Alzheimer A. On peculiar disease of the cerebral cortex. Allg Z Psychiatrie 1907:64:146

Alzheimer A. Über eigenartige Krankheitsfälle des späteren Alters. Z Gesamte Neurol Psychiatr 1911:4:356-385

Brun A. Frontal lobe degeneration of non-Alzheimer type. I. Neuropathology. Arch Gerontol Geriatr 1987:6:193-208

Baker M, MacKenzie IR, Pickering-Brown SM et al. Mutations in progranulin cause tau-negative frontotemporal dementia linked to chromosome 17. Nature. 2006 July16 (online publication)

Caselli RJ, Windebank AJ, Petersen RC, Komori T, Parisi JE, Okazaki H, Kokmen EM, Iverson Dinapoli RRP, Graff-Radford NR, and Stein SD. Rapidly progressive aphasic dementia and motor neuron disease. Ann Neurol 1993:33:200-207

Dubois B, Slachevsky A, Litvan I, and Pillon B. The FAB - A frontal assessment battery at bedside. Neurology 2000:55:1621-1626

Geschwind DH, Robidoux J, Alarcón M, Miller BL, Wilhelmsen KC, Cummings JL, and Nasreddine ZS. Dementia and neurodevelopmental predisposition: Cognitive dysfunction in presymptomatic subjects precedes dementia by decades in frontotemporal dementia. Ann Neurol 2001:50:741-746

Hutton M, et al. Association of missense and 5'-splice-site mutations in tau with the inherited dementia FTDP-17. Nature,1998;393:702-705

Hodges JR, Davies R, Xuereb J, Kril J, and Halliday G. Survival in frontotemporal dementia. Neurology 2003:61:349-354

Hodges JR, Patterson K, Oxbury S, and Funnell E. Semantic dementia: Progressive fluent aphasia with temporal lobe atrophy. Brain 1992:115:1783-1806

Jackson M, Lennox G, and Lowe J. Motor neurone disease-inclusion dementia. Neurodegeneration 1996:5:339-350

Kertesz A, Davidson W, and Fox H. Frontal Behavioral Inventory: Diagnostic criteria for Frontal Lobe Dementia. Can J Neurol Sci 1997:24:29-36

Kertesz A, Hillis A, and Munoz DG. Frontotemporal dementia and Pick's disease. Ann Neurol 54 Supplement 2003:5:S1-S35

Kertesz A, Hudson L, Mackenzie IR, and Munoz DG. The pathology and nosology of primary progressive aphasia. Neurology 1994:44:2065-2072

Kertesz A, Kawarai T, Rogaeva E, St.George-Hyslop PH, Poorkaj P, Bird TD, and Munoz DG. Familial frontotemporal dementia with ubiquitin-positive, tau-negative inclusions. Neurology 2000:54:818-827

Lebert F, Pasquier F. Trazodone in the treatment of behaviour in fronto-temporal dementia. Hum. Psychopharmacol Clin Exp 1999;14:279-281

Lomen-Hoerth C, Anderson T and Miller B. The overlap of amyotrophic lateral sclerosis and frontotemporal dementia. Neurology 2002:59:1077-1079

Mesulam M-M. Slowly progressive aphasia without generalized dementia. Ann Neurol 1982.11:592-598

Miller BL, Seeley WW, Mychack P, Rosen HJ, Mena I, and Boone K. Neuroanatomy of the self-evidence from patients with frontotemporal dementia. Neurology 2001:57:817-821

Miller BL, Cummings J, Mishin F, et al. Emergence of artistic talent in frontotemporal dementia. Neurology. 1998; 51:978-982

Mitsuyama Y. Presenile dementia with motor neuron disease in Japan: Clinicopathological review of 26 cases. J Neurol Neurosurg Psychiatry 1984:47:953-959

Munoz DG, Dickson DW, Bergeron C, Mackenzie IRA, Delacourte, and Zhukareva V. The neuropathology and biochemistry of frontotemporal dementia. Ann Neurol 2003:54 Suppl 5:S24-S28

Neary D, Snowden JS, Mann DMA, Northen B, Goulding PJ, and Macdermott N. Frontal lobe dementia and motor neuron disease. J Neurol Neurosurg Psychiatry 1990:53:23-32

Neary D, Snowden JS, Northen B, and Goulding P. Dementia of frontal lobe type. J Neurol Neurosurg Psychiatry 1988:51:353-361

Okamoto K, Hirai S, Yamazaki T, Sun X, and Nakazato Y. New ubiqui-tin-positive intraneuronal inclusions in the extra-motor cortices in patients with amyotrophic lateral sclerosis. Neurosci Lett 1991:129:233-236

Onari K and Spatz H. Anatomische Beitrage zur Lehre von der Pickschen umschriebenen Grosshirnrinden-Atrophie ("Picksche Krankheit""). Z Gesamte Neurol Psych 1926:101:470-511

Pick A. Über die Beziehungen der senilen Hirnatrophie zur Aphasie. Prag Med Wochenschr 1892:17:165-167

Pick A. Über primäre progressive Demenz bei Erwachsene. Prag Med Wochenschr 1904:29:417-420

Pick A. Uber einen weiteren Symptomenkomplex im Rahmen der Dementia senilis, bedingt durch umschriebene starkere Hirnatrophie (gemischte Apraxie). Monatsschr Psychiatr Neurologie 1906:19:97-108

Ratnaavalli E, Brayne C, Dawson K, and Hodges JR. The prevalence of frontotemporal dementia. Neurology 2002:58:1615-1621

Rebeiz JJ,.Kolodny EH, and Richardson EP, Jr. Corticodentatonigral degeneration with neuronal achromasia. Arch Neurol 1968:18:20-33

Rice GPA, Paty DW, Ball MJ, Tatham R, and A. Kertesz. Spongiform encephalopathy of long duration: A family study. Can J Neurol Sci 1980:7:171-174

Snowden JS, Bathgate D, Varma A, Blackshaw A, Gibbons ZC, and Neary D. Distinct behavioural profiles in frontotemporal dementia and semantic dementia. J Neurol Neurosurg Psychiatry 2001:70:323-332

Snowden JS, Goulding PJ, and Neary D. Semantic dementia: a form of circumscribed cerebral atrophy. Behav Neurol 1989:2:167-182

Snowden JS, Neary D, and Mann DMA. Fronto-Temporal Lobar Degeneration: Fronto-temporal Dementia, Progressive Aphasia, semantic dementia, London:Churchill Livingstone, 1996.

Sparks DL & Markesbery WR. Altered serotonergic and cholinergic synaptic markers in Pick's disease. Arch neurol 1991:48:796-799

Steele JC, Richardson JC, and Olszewski J. Progressive supranuclear palsy. Arch Neurol 1964:10:333-359

Swartz JR, Miller BL, Lesser IM, and Darby AL. Frontotemporal dementia: Treatment response to serotonin selective reuptake inhibitors. J Clin Psychiatry 1997:58:212-216

Tulving E. Episodic and semantic memory. In: Organization of memory, edited by E. Tulving and W. Donaldson, New York: Academic Press, 1972: p. 381-403

Warrington EK. The selective impairment of semantic memory. Quart J Exp Psych 27:635-657, 1975

Wernicke C. Einige neurere Arbeiten über Aphasie (Some new work on aphasia). Fortschritte der Medizin 1885:3:824, 4, pp. 377, 463

Wilhelmsen KC, Lynch T, Pavlou E, Higgins M, and Nygaard TG. Localization of disinhibition dementia parkinsonism amyotrophy complex to 17q21-22. Am J Hum Genet 1994:55:1159-1165

Zhukareva V. et al. Loss of tau defines novel sporadic and familial tauopathies with frontotemporal dementia. Ann. Neurol. 2001;49:165-175

ISBN 142510126-7

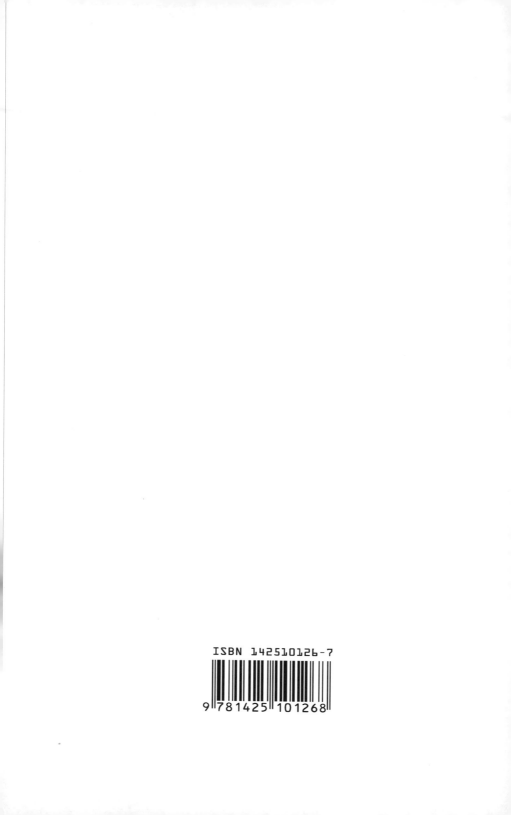

Made in the USA
San Bernardino, CA
03 March 2014